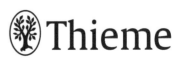

Facial Danger Zones

Staying Safe with Surgery, Fillers, and Non-Invasive Devices

Rod J. Rohrich, MD, FACS
Founding Professor and Chair
Department of Plastic Surgery
Distinguished Teaching Professor
UT Southwestern Medical Center
Founding Partner
Dallas Plastic Surgery Institute
Dallas, Texas

James M. Stuzin, MD
Plastic Surgeon
Institute of Aesthetic Medicine
Chair
Baker-Gordon Cosmetic Surgery Meeting
Professor of Plastic Surgery (Voluntary)
University of Miami School of Medicine
Miami, Florida

Erez Dayan, MD
Harvard Trained Plastic Surgeon
Dallas Plastic Surgery Institute
Dallas, Texas

E. Victor Ross, MD
Director
Scripps Clinic Laser and Cosmetic Dermatology Center
Scripps Clinic Carmel Valley
San Diego, California

Illustrations by Amanda Tomasikiewicz, CMI

Thieme
New York • Stuttgart • Delhi • Rio de Janeiro

Executive Editor: Sue Hodgson
Managing Editor: Nikole Y. Connors
Director, Editorial Services: Mary Jo Casey
Production Editor: Sean Woznicki
Illustrator: Amanda Tomasikiewicz
International Production Director: Andreas Schabert
Editorial Director: Sue Hodgson
International Marketing Director: Fiona Henderson
International Sales Director: Louisa Turrell
Director of Institutional Sales: Adam Bernacki
Senior Vice President and Chief Operating
  Officer: Sarah Vanderbilt
President: Brian D. Scanlan

Library of Congress Cataloging-in-Publication Data
Names: Rohrich, Rod J., author.
Title: Facial danger zones : staying safe with surgery, fillers,
  andnon-invasive devices / Rod J. Rohrich, MD, FACS, Founding
  Professor and Chair, Department of Plastic Surgery,
  Distinguished Teaching Professor, UT Southwestern
  Medical Center, Founding Partner, Dallas Plastic Surgery
  Institute, Dallas, Texas, James M. Stuzin, MD, Plastic Surgeon,
  Institute of Aesthetic Medicine, Chair of the Baker-Gordon
  Cosmetic Surgery meeting, Professor of Plastic Surgery
  (Voluntary), University of Miami School of Medicine, Miami,
  Florida, Erez Dayan, MD, Plastic Surgeon, Dallas Plastic Surgery
  Institute, Dallas, Texas, E. Victor Ross, MD, Director, Scripps
  Clinic Laser and Cosmetic Dermatology Center, Scripps Clinic
  Carmel Valley, San Diego, California.
Description: First edition. | New York: Thieme, [2019] | Summary:
  "The goal of this book is three-fold: - Optimal knowledge of
  facial anatomy is germane to obtaining the best results and safe
  outcomes in facial aesthetic surgery. This is especially the case
  with the intricate anatomy of the facial nerve in facelift surgery
  as discussed by Dr. James Stuzin. - Refine and define your
  knowledge on the vascular anatomy of the face to stay safe when
  performing facial fillers to prevent dreaded complications
  including blindness and skin loss, as discussed by
  Dr. Rod Rohrich. - Define the limitations and safety areas for the
  use of laser and minimally invasive technology from laser to
  Radiofrequency to ultrasound technology to optimize results
  and maximize safety in the face and neck areas as discussed by
  Dr. Erez Dayan and Dr. Vic Ross"– Provided by publisher.
Identifiers: LCCN 2019021417 (print) | LCCN 2019981257
  (ebook) | ISBN 9781684200030 | ISBN 9781684200047 (ebook)
Subjects: LCSH: Surgery, Plastic—Safety measures. | Face—Surgery. |
  Facial bones. | Lasers in surgery. | Face—Laser surgery.
Classification: LCC RD119.5.F33 R64 2019 (print) | LCC RD119.5.F33
  (ebook) | DDC 617.5/20592—dc23
LC record available at https://
  lccn.loc.gov/2019021417
LC ebook record available at https://
  lccn.loc.gov/2019981257

© 2020 Thieme Medical Publishers, Inc.

Thieme Publishers New York
333 Seventh Avenue, New York, NY 10001 USA
+1 800 782 3488, customerservice@thieme.com

Thieme Publishers Stuttgart
Rüdigerstrasse 14, 70469 Stuttgart, Germany
+49 [0]711 8931 421, customerservice@thieme.de

Thieme Publishers Delhi
A-12, Second Floor, Sector-2, Noida-201301
Uttar Pradesh, India
+91 120 45 566 00, customerservice@thieme.in

Thieme Publishers Rio de Janeiro, Thieme Publicações Ltda.
Edifício Rodolpho de Paoli, 25º andar
Av. Nilo Peçanha, 50 – Sala 2508,
Rio de Janeiro 20020-906 Brasil
+55 21 3172-2297 / +55 21 3172-1896
www.thiemerevinter.com.br

Cover design: Thieme Publishing Group
Typesetting by DiTech Process Solutions

Printed in Germany by Beltz Grafische Betriebe   9 8 7 6 5

ISBN 978-1-68420-003-0

Also available as an e-book:
eISBN 978-1-68420-004-7

Important note: Medicine is an ever-changing science undergoing continual development. Research and clinical experience are continually expanding our knowledge, in particular our knowledge of proper treatment and drug therapy. Insofar as this book mentions any dosage or application, readers may rest assured that the authors, editors, and publishers have made every effort to ensure that such references are in accordance with **the state of knowledge at the time of production of the book.**

Nevertheless, this does not involve, imply, or express any guarantee or responsibility on the part of the publishers in respect to any dosage instructions and forms of applications stated in the book. **Every user is requested to examine carefull**y the manufacturers' leaflets accompanying each drug and to check, if necessary in consultation with a physician or specialist, whether the dosage schedules mentioned therein or the contraindications stated by the manufacturers differ from the statements made in the present book. Such examination is particularly important with drugs that are either rarely used or have been newly released on the market. Every dosage schedule or every form of application used is entirely at the user's own risk and responsibility. The authors and publishers request every user to report to the publishers any discrepancies or inaccuracies noticed. If errors in this work are found after publication, errata will be posted at www.thieme.com on the product description page.

Some of the product names, patents, and registered designs referred to in this book are in fact registered trademarks or proprietary names even though specific reference to this fact is not always made in the text. Therefore, the appearance of a name without designation as proprietary is not to be construed as a representation by the publisher that it is in the public domain.

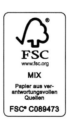

Contents

Contents

Video Contents

Preface

Why a new book on FACIAL DANGER ZONES? We would like to share our thoughts why we felt a new contribution to the literature on this topic was appropriate at this time.

The key textbook was written over 20 years ago by Dr. Brooke Seckel, who is unique in being both a board-certified neurologist as well as a plastic surgeon. Dr Seckel noted that what motivated him to write the first edition was his concern regarding the potential for facial nerve injuries following the more aggressive sub-SMAS face lift procedures described in the early 1990s. His textbook went on to become a go-to reference for surgeons performing both reconstructive and anesthetic facial procedures in that era and was republished in 2010 for the next generation of plastic surgeons.

Over the last decade much has changed in the world of aesthetic surgery and cosmetic medicine. The growth in global demand for aesthetic procedures advances at a rapid rate and with this growth comes an increasing mandate for patient safety. Aesthetic procedures now encompass both surgical and nonsurgical techniques and are performed by physicians from many disciples. We have noted with increasing demand comes new and more distressing complications. Blindness following injectable fillers was unheard of when Dr Seckel wrote the FACIAL DANGER ZONES, but now is reported with unfortunate frequency. Plastic surgery residencies commonly stress reconstructive procedures, while facial anatomy is more superficially taught and little time is spent on the nuances of facial aesthetic procedures. We have noted our residents seem more comfortable executing a complex microvasular reconstruction than performing a facelift, and physicians are too commonly offering procedures to their patients that were not well taught during their training. Twenty years after the initial publication of this textbook, the increasing need for patient safety remains paramount, leading to our interest in redefining the state-of-the-art in FACIAL DANGER ZONES.

While techniques have changed and the delivery of care has evolved among the many specialties preforming aesthetic procedures, anatomy remains constant. From our perspective, it is the three-dimensional knowledge of both facial soft tissue anatomy as well as vascular anatomy that remains the key to avoiding complications such as motor branch injury, blindness and tissue ischemia. The proliferation of non-invasive devices and lasers also mandates an understanding of the safety consideration and limitations when utilizing these devices.

The goal of this book is three-fold:

- Optimal knowledge of facial anatomy is germane to obtaining the best results and safe outcomes in facial aesthetic surgery. This is especially the case with the intricate anatomy of the facial nerve in facelift surgery as discussed by Dr. James Stuzin.
- Refine and define your knowledge on the vascular anatomy of the face to stay safe when performing facial fillers to prevent dreaded complications including blindness and skin loss, as discussed by Dr. Rod Rohrich.
- Define the limitations and safety areas for the use of laser and minimally invasive technology from laser to Radiofrequency to ultrasound technology to optimize results and maximize safety in the face and neck areas as discussed by Dr. Erez Dayan and Dr. Vic Ross.

In writing FACIAL DANGER ZONES we went back to the cadaver lab to ensure that the anatomy presented is accurate and that the complexities of facial soft tissue anatomy become demystified. We have included the critical cadaver photos required to clarify anatomy combined with artists illustrations and short video vignettes in the hope that the reader will easily understand a subject that we feel has been made overly complicated in the literature. The format of the book is to streamline this knowledge and with the addition of video and a digital e-book copy it is our sincere hope that the physician can go directly from this textbook into the operating room or treatment room and preform aesthetic procedures with both greater confidence and safety.

The responsibility of physicians preforming cosmetic medicine procedures remains precision in outcomes and patient safety. While artistry in cosmetic medicine is both visual and intuitive, the analytical basis for consistency is a fundamental and thorough knowledge of anatomy and its relationship to facial shape. It is our sincere hope that this textbook provides the reader with the basis for a solid three-dimensional understanding of facial soft tissue anatomy and an awareness of the danger zones when performing procedures, leading to safe and satisfying results for both patients and physicians.

Rod J. Rohrich, MD
James M. Stuzin, MD
Erez Dayan, MD
E. Victor Ross, MD

Dedication/Acknowledgements

We dedicate this patient book to the safety of all our patients. We hope that this work helps clinicians focus on safety. Consumers can use this book to guide them to the best board certified Plastic Surgeons, Dermatologists, Facial Plastic Surgeons, and Oculoplastic Surgeons that will provide them with best care based upon the principles we have delineated in this book.

Cosmetic surgery is all about putting your patient and their safety & outcome first and foremost. This book highlights this need and mandates that we all have a responsibility as physicians to do no harm.

We also acknowledge and appreciate all our patients who have helped each of us become better and more caring physicians throughout our practice of medicine.

Specifically, we want to thank our individual staff that have helped us complete this book, including Diane Sinn my long term assistant and administrator, and our great Thieme staff Judith Tomat and our publisher Sue Hodgson as well as our illustrator Amanda Tomasikiewicz whose expertise is displayed in each page of this wonderful book.

Sincerely,

Rod J. Rohrich, MD
James M. Stuzin, MD
Erez Dayan, MD
E. Victor Ross, MD

Contributors

Erez Dayan, MD
Harvard Trained Plastic Surgeon
Dallas Plastic Surgery Institute
Dallas, Texas

Raja Mohan, MD
Accent on You Plastic Surgery
Arlington, Texas

Rod J. Rohrich, MD, FACS
Founding Professor and Chair
Department of Plastic Surgery
Distinguished Teaching Professor
UT Southwestern Medical Center
Founding Partner
Dallas Plastic Surgery Institute
Dallas, Texas

E. Victor Ross, MD
Director
Scripps Clinic Laser and Cosmetic Dermatology Center
Scripps Clinic Carmel Valley
San Diego, California

James M. Stuzin, MD
Plastic Surgeon
Institute of Aesthetic Medicine
Chair of the Baker-Gordon Cosmetic Surgery Meeting
Professor of Plastic Surgery (Voluntary)
University of Miami School of Medicine
Miami, Florida

David Dwayne Weir, MNS, APRN, NP-C
Dallas Plastic Surgery Institute
Dallas, Texas

Dinah Wan, MD
Southlake Plastic Surgery
Southlake, Texas

Part I

Facial Nerves

James M. Stuzin

1 Overview of Facial Tissue Anatomy

James M. Stuzin

Abstract

The key to safety in surgical dissection of the face is an accurate understanding of soft tissue anatomy. While two-dimensional branching patterns of the facial nerve are variable, the plane of the facial nerve is constant within the architecture of the facial soft tissue. Recognition of the plane of surgical dissection and its relationship to the plane of the facial nerve provides the surgeon with the ability to provide safe and consistent outcomes in both aesthetic and reconstructive facial procedures.

Keywords: facial soft tissue anatomy, facial nerve

The primary focus of this textbook is to assist physicians operating within the face to improve their understanding of the nuances of facial anatomy, increasing both consistency in result and patient safety. Understanding facial soft-tissue anatomy is pertinent to both reconstructive and aesthetic surgery, and a three-dimensional comprehension of the architectural arrangement of facial soft tissue is essential when dissecting facial flaps for reconstructive purposes or performing procedures to expose the craniofacial skeleton, and more specifically when performing aesthetic surgery procedures.

Preventing facial nerve injury is the most important aspect of both safety and preserving function when performing facial procedures. The critical element to avoid motor branch injury is an accurate understanding of the three-dimensional architecture of facial soft tissue.

While much has been written about facial nerve anatomy, many investigations have focused on two-dimensional branching patterns of the facial nerve. Unfortunately, two-dimensional facial nerve anatomy is not particularly relevant when dissecting within the face, as there is a great deal of variation in terms of branching patterns among patients as well as variations in branching patterns between the right and left side of the cheek. The key to avoiding facial nerve injury is to understand the three-dimensional architecture of the soft tissue planes of the face, as well as recognizing the plane of dissection in relation to the plane of the facial nerve. THINK THREE DIMENSIONALLY.

1.1 The Architectural Arrangement of Facial Soft Tissue

- Facial soft tissue is arranged in a series of concentric layers, similar to the concentric layers of an onion.

1.1.1 The Layers of Facial Soft Tissue from Superficial to Deep

- Skin
- Compartmentalized subcutaneous fat
- Superficial facial fascia (also termed SMAS; these terms will be used interchangeably)
- Mimetic muscles (superficial muscles invested by the SMAS)
- Subsmas fat
- Deep facial fascia (also regionally known as parotid capsule, masseteric fascia, or deep temporal fascia)
- The plane of the facial nerve, parotid duct, and buccal fat pad (▶ **Fig. 1.1a,b**).

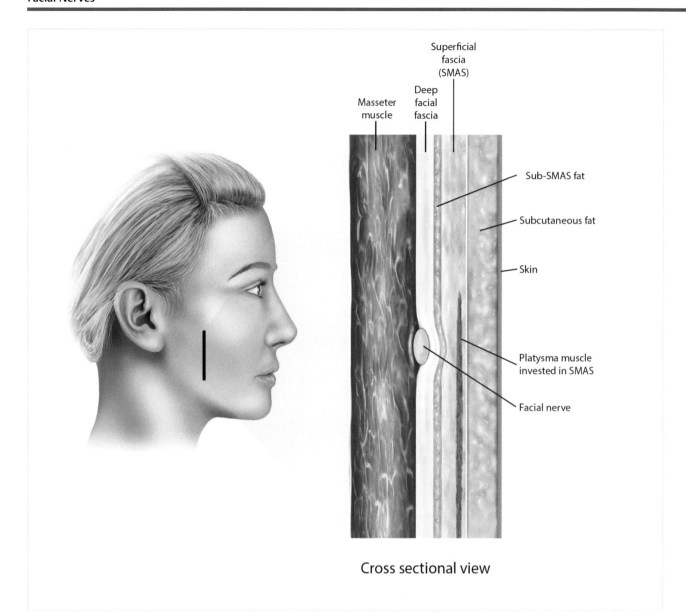

Cross sectional view

Fig. 1.1 (a) Cross section of the lateral cheek illustrated just anterior to the parotid gland. The architecture of the facial soft tissues of the cheek is three-dimensional and is arranged in a series of concentric layers. From superficial to deep, these layers are 1) skin 2) subcutaneous fat (which is compartmentalized) 3) superficial facial fascia-better know as SMAS 4) superficial mimetic muscles (invested by SMAS) 5) sub-Smas fat 6) deep facial fascia (also regionally termed parotid capsule, masseteric fascia, or deep temporal fascia 7) the plane of facial nerve, parotid duct, masseter, and buccal fat pad. The KEY to SAFETY when operating in the face is to recognize the plane of dissection and its relation to the plane of the facial nerve.

1.1.2 The Plane of the Facial Nerve

- While there is a good deal of variation in terms of two-dimensional facial nerve branching patterns, the plane of the facial nerve in relation to the other fascia layers of the face is anatomically constant.
- The critical step to avoid facial nerve injury is to accurately identify the plane of dissection as it is performed. If dissection is carried out either superficially or deeply to the plane of the facial nerve, motor branch injury will be prevented.

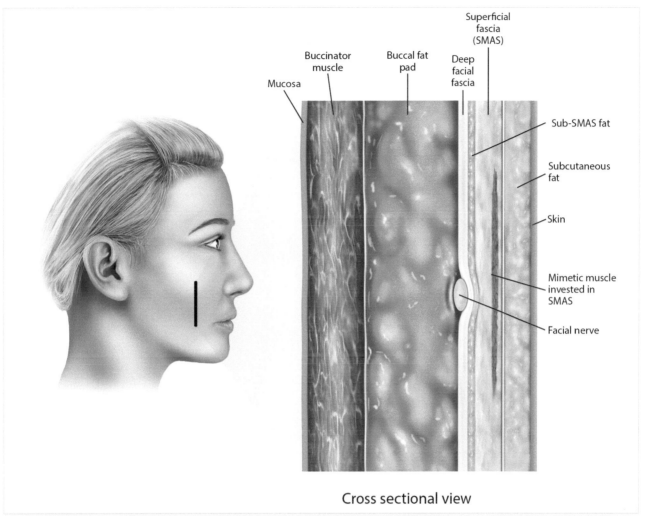

Cross sectional view

Fig. 1.1 (b) Cross section of the soft tissue of the midcheek, just anterior to the masseter and overlying the buccal fat pad. The concentric architecture of soft tissue is similar to the lateral cheek, though the facial nerve branches tend to become more superficial as they travel toward the muscles they innervate. Note that in this region of the cheek, the buccal fat pad and facial nerve branches lie in the same plane, just deep to the deep fascia. More anteriorly, the facial nerve branches penetrate the deep fascia and innervate mimetic muscles along their deep surfaces.

- While the plane of the facial nerve is constant from patient to patient, both the thickness and the appearance of each anatomic layer varies significantly, such that the nuance of plane identification becomes the key to safe dissection.
- Just as skin thickness varies from patient to patient, so does the thickness of the underlying subcutaneous fat and SMAS. Similarly, the presence or absence of sub-SMAS fat, and the thickness of the underlying glistening deep facial fascia will appear different in many patients.
- Typically, these layers are better defined and thicker in younger patients than in in older patients. Similarly, reoperative surgery or reconstructive procedures following trauma can distort the appearance of fascial planes. Nonetheless, the architectural arrangement remains constant and is present in all patients, and the key to safety for the surgeon is to recognize what plane is being dissected when operating within the face. (see **Video 1.1**).

1.1.3 Layers of Facial Soft Tissue

Skin

- The skin's thickness and vascularity vary from patient to patient.
- When performing a facelift or raising a cervicofacial flap for facial reconstruction, the key to safety is to perform the dissection within the underlying subcutaneous fat, superficial to the SMAS.
- The use of transillumination to define the interface between the subcutaneous fat and the superficial fascia is helpful in defining the correct plane of dissection (▶Fig. 1.2, **Video 1.2**).

Subcutaneous Fat

- The plane of the subcutaneous fat is the dissection plane typically utilized in both reconstructive and aesthetic facial procedures and is anatomically situated as an interposition between the skin dissection and the underlying superficial fascia (SMAS).
- Facial subcutaneous fat is not a homogenous structure, but is separated into a series of separate "facial fat compartments."
- The fibrous septa, which separate the subcutaneous fat into compartments, represent the distal ramifications of the retaining ligaments, which travel from deep fixed structures such as the parotid gland to penetrate the SMAS and inset into the overlying skin.
- Vascular perforators similarly transit from deep to superficial adjacent to the retaining ligaments, such that as dissection proceeds from one

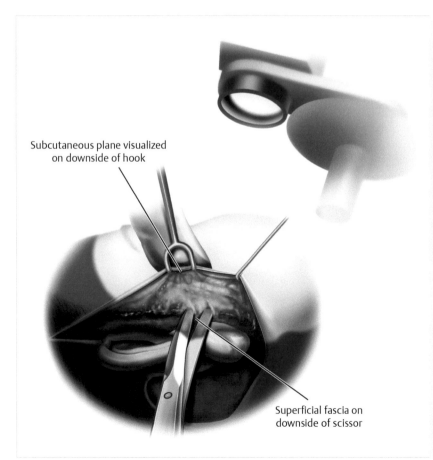

Subcutaneous plane visualized on downside of hook

Superficial fascia on downside of scissor

Fig. 1.2 Transillumination utilizing light from the opposite side of the patient is useful in defining the interface between the subcutaneous fat and the SMAS and adds greater precision to subcutaneous dissection in terms of controlling skin-flap thickness. While blunt subcutaneous dissection in general is safe, in thin patients with little subcutaneous fat or in reoperative surgery, utilizing transillumination is helpful for accurate plane dissection (see video clip as well).

compartment to an adjoining facial fat compartment, bleeding from these perforators is noted.

- Both the thickness and fascial consistency of the fat within each compartment varies as the cheek is dissected, from laterally in the preauricular region more anteriorly toward the nasolabial fold.
    - The lateral compartment, in the preauricular region, tends to be thin, dense, and vascular, while the fat within the middle compartment tends to be thick, fluffy, avascular, and easy to dissect.
    - Transiting from the middle to the malar compartment, zygomatic ligaments and perforators from the transverse facial artery are encountered such that dissection along the lateral malar eminence tends to be both fibrous and bloody.
- Each facial fat compartment has its own tendency toward deflation, with the lateral compartments showing evidence of deflation in patients in the 40 to 50 year age group, while malar deflation tends to occur a decade later. The anatomic nature of deflation (which is compartment-specific) explains why facial deflation tends to occur regionally, rather than homogenously across the cheek in facial aging (See Chapter 2 on Facial Fat Compartments) (▶ **Fig. 1.3**).

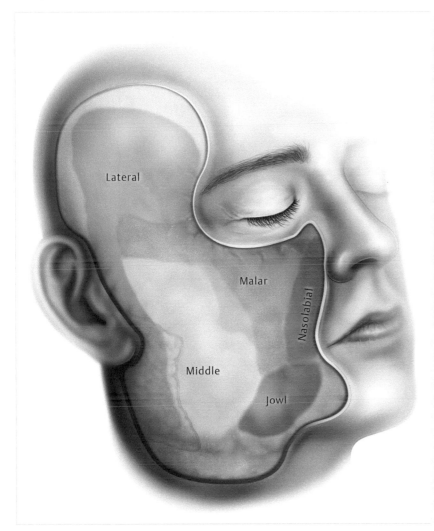

Fig. 1.3 Facial subcutaneous fat is not a homogeneous layer, which is dissimilar to subcutaneous fat in other regions of the body. The subcutaneous fat of the cheek is divided into fibrous compartments by the distal ramifications of the retaining ligaments as they transit from deep-fixed structures to insert into the skin as the retinacular cutis. The superficial compartments of the cheek (from lateral to medial) are the lateral compartment, middle compartment, malar compartment, jowl compartment, and nasolabial compartment. Each fat compartment has a distinct fascial consistency, thickness, and a specific tendency toward deflation with age.

SMAS (Superficial Facial Fascia)

- The SMAS represents the superficial facial fascia and is analogous to superficial fascia elsewhere in the body. It is continuous with the superficial cervical fascia in the neck and extends cephalically toward the scalp, forming a continuous fascial layer within the head and neck.
- The superficial fascia is intimately associated with the overlying facial subcutaneous fat and skin through the distal ramifications of the retaining ligaments known as the retinacula cutis. The SMAS, subcutaneous fat, and skin represent the mobile unit of the facial soft tissue, (as opposed to the deep fixed structures of the face).
- Many of the morphologic changes in facial shape result from a loss of support from the deep retaining ligaments, which allows this mobile unit of facial soft tissue to change its relation to deeply fixed facial structures, accounting for facial fat descent and radial expansion in aging.

Mimetic Muscles

- The muscles of facial expression, which produce movement of the overlying facial skin, are intimately associated with the superficial fascia, with the superficial fascia serving as the fibrous connection between muscle and skin.
- The anatomic relationship between the SMAS and mimetic muscles is termed investiture, which is defined as the superficial fascia (SMAS) lining both the superficial and deep surfaces of the mimetic muscle. Mimetic muscles invested by the SMAS are connected to the overlying skin by the fine fibers of the retinacular cutis, which allows muscular contraction to produce soft tissue and skin movement.
- From a surgical perspective, most mimetic muscles are situated superficial to the plane of the facial nerve. Resulting from these muscles' being situated superficial to the plane of the facial nerve, they receive their innervation along their deep surfaces.
- Only three mimetic muscles are situated deep to the plane of the facial nerve within the three-dimensional architecture of the facial soft tissue. These deeply-situated muscles include the levator anguli oris, the mentalis, and the buccinator. As these three muscles lie deep to the plane of the facial nerve, their innervation occurs along their superficial surfaces (▶ Fig. 1.4).
- The surgical significance of the anatomic relationship between the depth of the mimetic muscle and its innervation is relevant to prevention of facial nerve injury. As most mimetic muscles receive innervation along their deep surfaces, when encountering a mimetic muscle during surgical dissection, carrying the dissection along the superficial surface of this muscles will prevent a motor branch injury.
  - For example, when encountering the platysma in the lower cheek and neck, dissecting superficial to the platysma will prevent injury to both the cervical and marginal mandibular nerve branches, which travel deep to this muscle.
  - Similarly, when dissecting in the malar region, dissecting superficial to the orbicularis oculi, and zygomaticus major and minor will preserve muscular innervation, as these muscles are innervated along their deep surfaces (▶ Fig. 1.5).

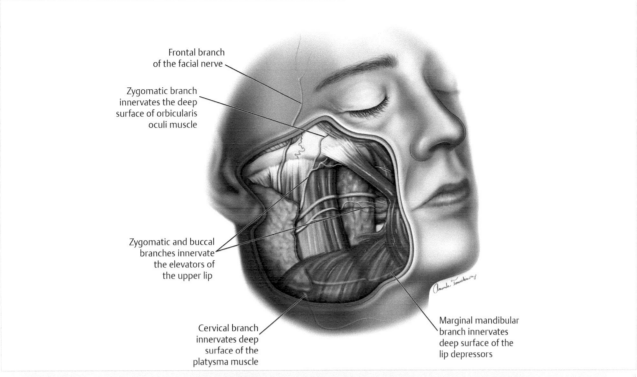

Frontal branch
of the facial nerve

Zygomatic branch
innervates the deep
surface of orbicularis
oculi muscle

Zygomatic and buccal
branches innervate
the elevators of
the upper lip

Cervical branch
innervates deep
surface of the
platysma muscle

Marginal mandibular
branch innervates
deep surface of the
lip depressors

Fig. 1.4 Mimetic muscles are situated at different levels within the facial soft tissue, with muscles such as the orbicularis oculi situated directly beneath the skin (producing crow's feet in animation with aging) while deeply-situated muscles, such as the bucccinator, overlie oral mucosa. As most of the mimetic muscles lie superficial to the plane of the facial nerve, they receive their innervation along their deep surfaces. For this reason, if dissection is carried along the superficial surface of a mimetic muscle (i.e., superficial to the platysma in the cheek and neck), motor branch injury will be prevented.

In general, the facial nerve branches lie deep to the deep fascia until reaching the muscles, which they innervate. They then penetrate the deep fascia to innervate the muscle along its deep surface. The exceptions to this are the frontal and cervical branches. In this illustration, the deep fascia has been removed to demonstrate the depth of nerve branches in relation to the muscles, which are innervated.

Note that the cervical branch typically penetrates the deep fascia laterally and lies with the plane between superficial and deep fascia, just deep to the platysma, before innervating the platysma medially. Similarly, the frontal branch travels in the plane between superficial and deep fascia after it travels cephalad to the zygomatic arch.

Deep Facial Fascia

- Similar to the SMAS, the deep facial fascia represents a continuation of deep cervical fascia cephalad into the face and is anatomically similar to deep fascia elsewhere in the body.
- Despite existing as a continuous layer, regional variations of deep fascia have been given specific nomenclature. Overlying the parotid, the deep fascia is termed parotid capsule; overlying the masseter, the deep fascia is termed masseteric fascia; and in the temporal region, it is commonly termed deep temporal fascia.
- THE IMPORTANT POINT TO REMEMBER IS THAT ALL FACIAL NERVE BRANCHES WITHIN THE CHEEK LIE DEEP TO THE DEEP FACIAL FASCIA AFTER THEY EXIT THE PAROTID.
- Therefore, as long as the dissection is kept superficial to the deep fascia, motor branch injury will be prevented in most regions of the cheek. From an anatomic perspective, it is the presence of the deep fascia that

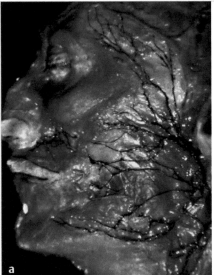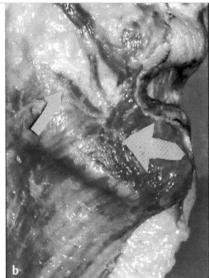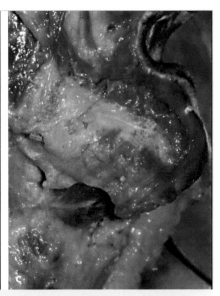

Fig. 1.5 **(a)** Cadaver dissection of the facial nerve (performed by Dr. Julia Terzis). Note that the malar region, directly overlying the zygomatic eminence, is a watershed between the frontal branches superiorly and the zygomatic branches inferiorly, such that dissection directly overlying the malar eminence is safe in terms of inadvertent nerve injury. Note also that the elevators of the upper lip receive their innervation along their deep surfaces, such that dissection along the superficial surface of these muscles is similarly safe.

(*From Surgical Rejuvenation of the Face. Baker, Gordon and Stuzin in 1996 published by Mosby*) **(b)** The mimetic muscles that might be encountered when performing dissection in the cheek are shown in this cadaver dissection. They include the zygomaticus major (which sends a slip of muscle to the modiolus), the risorius (*small arrow*), the platysma, the depressor anguli oris (*large arrow*), and the depressor inferioris. Note the relative size of the platysma in comparison to the other depressors of the lower lip. While the platysma does not have a direct insertion into the lip, its function for full denture smile and animation is important. These muscles are interrelated in terms of function by connections, which exist between the cervical and marginal nerves.

(*From Lambros, V, Stuzin, JM, The Cross-Cheek Depression: Surgical Cause and Effect in the Development of the "Joker Line" and its Treatment. Plast Reconst Surg. 122:1543, 2008*)

(c) The depressor angli oris and depressor inferioris are reflected to demonstrate the marginal mandibular nerve, which innervates these muscles along their deep surfaces.

allows sub-SMAS dissection to proceed safely, as the deep fascia serves as an interposition layer between sub-SMAS dissection and the underlying facial nerve branches (▶ **Fig. 1.6**).

Facial Nerve, Parotid Duct, and Buccal Fat Pad

- Deep to the deep fascia lies the plane of the facial nerve, parotid duct, and buccal fat pad.
- Obviously, this is a plane that is to be avoided during soft tissue dissection of the cheek.
- Deep to the plane of the facial nerve are situated the fixed structures of the face, including the parotid gland, masseter, deep fat compartments, and periosteum.

1.1.4 Retaining Ligaments

- Retaining ligaments of the cheek support the facial soft tissue against gravitational change and exist in specific locations.
- These ligaments originate deep to the deep fascia and travel from deep fixed structure, through the SMAS, and insert into the overlying skin via the retinacular cutis.

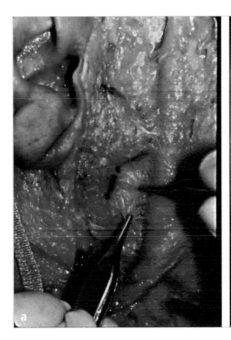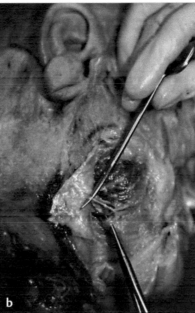

Fig. 1.6 **(a)** illustrates the surgical separation of the superficial and deep fascia, exposing the parotid capsule and masseteric fascia. **(b)** demonstrates that the facial nerve branches in the cheek situated deep to the deep fascia, such that sub-SMAS dissection of the cheek is safe as long as the dissection proceeds superficial to the deep fascia. Recognition of the plane of dissection and its relation to the plane of the facial nerve is the key element to preventing facial nerve injury. *(From Stuzin, JM, Baker, TJ, Gordon, HL: The relationship of the superficial and deep facial fascias: relevance to rhytidectomy and aging. Plast Reconstr Surg, 89:441 1992)*

- Each series of ligaments is named based on the anatomic location of the fibers.
  - Those ligaments originating from attachments to the parotid gland (both the main and accessory lobes) are termed parotid cutaneous ligaments, supporting the soft tissues of the lateral cheek.
  - Ligaments originating from the periosteum of lateral zygoma are termed zygomatic ligaments and support the upper and lateral cheek, fixating the malar fat pad to the lateral zygoma.
  - Ligaments originating along the anterior border of the masseter are termed masseteric cutaneous ligaments and support the mid and lower cheek and jowl fat.
  - Ligaments originating from the periosteum of the parasymphyseal and symphyseal region of the mandible are termed mandibular ligaments and support the soft-tissue chin pad to the underlying mandibular symphysis.
- Of surgical significance, ligaments will be encountered when performing both subcutaneous and sub-SMAS dissection.
  - In general, the sub-SMAS appearance of these ligaments tends to exhibit defined thick fibers, while superficial to the SMAS, the ligaments are thinner and more numerous as the retinacular cutis fans out to insert into cheek skin.
  - When dissecting either subcutaneously or in the sub-SMAS plane, ligament recognition, as well as identifying when the dissection has proceeded distal to the restraint of the retaining ligaments (into the mobile areas of the cheek), provides the surgeon a patient-specific anatomic destination for the degree of surgical release required for flap repositioning (▶**Fig. 1.7**).

Parotid Cutaneous Ligaments

- Parotid cutaneous ligaments are dense fibrous structures which support facial skin in the preauricular and lateral cheek to the underlying parotid capsule.

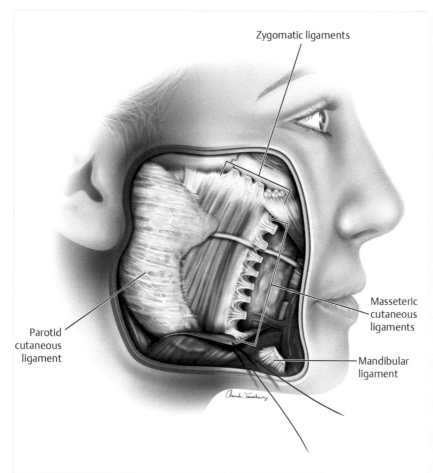

Zygomatic ligaments

Parotid cutaneous ligament

Masseteric cutaneous ligaments

Mandibular ligament

Fig. 1.7 The retaining ligaments of the cheek receive their origin from deep-fixed structures and then transit superficially through the SMAS to insert into the skin as the retinacular cutis. The ligaments of the cheek are 1) parotidocutaneous ligaments 2) zygomatic ligaments 3) masseteric ligaments 4) mandibular ligaments.
Not all ligaments are of the same density, and the parotidocutaneous, lateral zygomatic, and upper masseteric ligaments tend to be the stoutest fibers within the cheek.

- These ligaments are intimately associated with the lateral fat compartment in the preauricular region of the cheek and account for the fibrous and fascial quality of the subcutaneous dissection within the preauricular area.

Zygomatic Ligaments

- The zygomatic ligaments originate from the periosteum of the lateral zygoma and are dense and well-defined in the region where the zygomatic arch joins the lateral malar eminence, extending through the lateral malar region.
- The zygomatic ligaments tend to be thick, discrete fibers and are encountered both in the subcutaneous and sub-SMAS plane when dissecting over the lateral zygoma.
- From a surgical perspective, release of the lateral zygomtic ligaments in the subcutaneous plane improves skin flap redraping when mobilizing a cervicofacial skin flap.
- Similarly, release of the zygomatic ligaments in the sub-SMAS plane allows repositioning of the malar fat pad to restore lateral malar volumetric highlights. It is the anatomic repositioning of the malar pad which serves as the basis for extended SMAS and high SMAS techniques for facial rejuvenation (▶ **Fig. 1.8**).

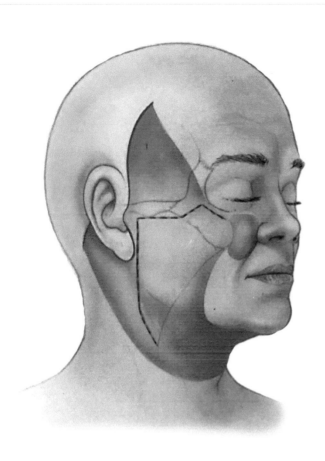

Fig. 1.8 An extended SMAS or high SMAS dissection releases the SMAS from the restraint of the partotidcutoneous ligaments, the lateral zygomatic ligaments, and the upper masseteric ligaments, allowing elevation of the malar fat pad (*shown in green*) and cheek fat superiorly to enhance facial shape in facelifting. While not all facial ligaments require surgical release for adequate flap mobility, dissection of the SMAS from the restraint of the stout ligaments along the parotid, lateral zygoma, and upper masseter remains a key element in terms of consistency for facial fat repositioning in facelifting.

Masseteric Ligaments

- The masseteric ligaments extend along the entire anterior border of the masseter. The most discreet and dense fibers are noted superiorly along the superior boarder of the masseter, where they blend with the inferior zygomatic ligaments.
- While the ligaments along the middle boarder of the masseter tend to be weak, the caudal masseteric ligaments are also discreet fibrous structures, binding the platysma and jowl fat to the caudal masseter in the region of the mandibular angle.

Mandibular Ligmaments

- Mandibular ligaments are noted along the parasymphyseal region of the mandible and more medially percolate through the soft-tissue chin pad, fixating the chin to the underlying mandibular symphysis.
- The mandibular ligaments are dense fibers which extend through the chin pad and extend caudally to insert along the caudal border of the mandibular symphysis.
- The caudal insertions of the mandibular ligaments are responsible for the formation of the submental crease in aging. On profile view in older patients, the submental crease demarcates the junction between the aging chin and the aging neck and anatomically is formed by a merging of the insertion of the medial platysma juxtaposed to the caudal insertion of the mandibular ligaments (►**Fig. 1.9**).

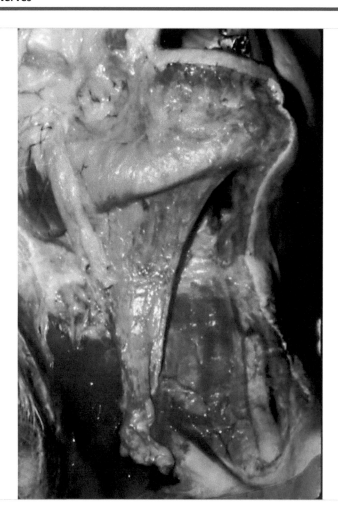

Fig. 1.9 The platysma insertion into the periosteum of the parasymphaseal region of the mandible and mandibular symphysis contributes to the formation of the mandibular ligaments, which support the soft-tissue chin pad in normal anatomic position in youth. The insertion of the platysma along the caudal symphysis contributes in aging to the formation of the submental crease, which delineates the aging chin from the aging neck.

Surgical Significance of the Retaining Ligaments

- The surgical significance of the retaining ligaments is that they delineate the degree of dissection required to mobilize both the skin and the SMAS in surgical rejuvenation of the aging face.
- In terms of skin-flap mobilization, the subcutaneous dissection required to proceed from the fixed lateral cheek anteriorly to the mobile region of the cheek requires dissection of the skin flap anterior to the restraint of the zygomatic ligaments as well as anterior to the masseter and adjoining masseteric ligaments.
- Regarding sub-SMAS mobilization, the SMAS laterally in the cheek is firmly adherent to the parotid, accessory lobe of the parotid, lateral zygoma, and the upper masseter, all of which represent regions of high ligamentous density.
- For this reason, to adequately release the SMAS requires that the SMAS be dissected from the parotid, accessory lobe of the parotid, lateral zygoma and the upper masseteric ligaments.
- Once the SMAS is released from these structures, the mobile region of the sub-SMAS within the anterior cheek is identified, and the dissection becomes less fibrous (see Chapter 8).
- In both skin and sub-SMAS dissection, once the dissection has proceeded past the restraint of the retaining ligaments, further anterior dissection does not improve soft-tissue movement and only serves to increase the

morbidity of the procedure. Recognition of the limits of required dissection as it proceeds past the retaining ligaments provides an individualized approach to flap mobilization which is patient specific, adding greater precision and consistency in post operative recovery and result.

1.2 Summary

Perhaps no other area of the body is as anatomically complex as the face, and from a surgical perspective, the risk of facial nerve injury can only be ameliorated if the nuances of soft-tissue anatomy are recognized. As facial nerve branching patterns are variable, the key to safety when operating within the cheek is to recognize the plane of the facial nerve and ensure that the surgical plane of dissection is carried superficial or deep to the plane of the nerve.

THINK THREE-DIMENSIONALLY, and RECOGNIZE THE PLANE OF DISSECTION WHEN OPERATING WITHIN THE CHEEK.

Suggested Readings

Baker DC, Conley, J: Avoiding facial nerve injuries in rhytidectomy: anatomic variations and pitfalls; Plast Reconstr Surg; 64:781, 1979.

Freilinger, G, Grube H, Happak W Pechmann, U: Surgical anatomy of the mimic muscle system and the facial nerve: importance for reconstructive and aesthetic surgery. Plast Reconstr Surg; 80:686, 1987.

Bosse JP, Papilloon, J. Sirgoca; anatomy of the SMAS at the malar region. In Maneksha, RJ. Ed. Transactions of the IX International Congress of Plastic and Reconstructive Surgery, New York, McGraw Hill, 1987.

Furnas D: The retaining ligaments of the cheek. Plast Reconstr Surg, 83:11, 1989.

Mendelson, BC, Wong, CH, Surgical Anatomy of the Middle Premasseter Space and its Application in Sub-SMAS Face lift Surgery. Plast Reconst Surg. 132:57, 2013.

Mendelson, BC, Muzaffar, A, Adams, W. Surgical Anatomy of the Midceek and Malar Mounds. Plast Reconstr Surg. 110:885, 2002.

Mendelson, BC, Jacobson, SR. Surgical anatomy of the midcheek: Facial layers, spaces and the midcheek segments. Clin plast Surg 2008:395, 2008

Mitz V, Peyonie, M: The superficial musculoaponeurotic system (SMAS) in the parotid and cheek area. Plast Reconstr Surg, 58:80, 1976.

Roostaeian, J. Rohrich, R. Stuzin, J. Anatomical Considerations to Prevent Facial Nerve Injury. Plast Reconstr. Surg. 135: 1318, 2015.

Seckel, B. Facial Nerve Danger Zones, 2nd edition. CRC Press, Boca Raton, Fl., 2010

Skoog, T: Plastic Surgery- New Methods and Refinements. Philadelphia, WB Saunders, 1974.

Stuzin, JM, Baker, TJ, Gordon, HL: The relationship of the superficial and deep facial fascias: relevance to rhytidectomy and aging. Plast Reconstr Surg, 89:441 1992..

Terzis, JK, Barmpitsioti, A. Essays on the Facial Nerve: Part I. Microanatomy. Plast Reconstr Surg. 125: 879, 2010.

2 Facial Fat Compartments

James M. Stuzin

Abstract

Facial fat differs from fat in other regions of the body as it is compartmentalized. Each facial fat compartment exhibits septal boundaries, a regional perforator blood supply, and a specific tendency toward deflation in aging.

Recognition of compartment anatomy is one of the keys to safe subcutaneous dissection of the cheek, as facial nerve branches are often superficially positioned at transition points between compartments. Recognition of compartment-specific deflation provides a guideline for volume restoration in facial rejuvenation.

Keywords: facial fat compartments, facial deflation

Key Points

- Subcutaneous facial fat is not homogeneous but rather partitioned into a series of compartments separated by specific fibrous septa.
- Each facial fat compartment has its own vascular blood supply, thickness and fascial consistency.
- Some fat compartments are thin and fibrous, while others typically contain a large volume of easily dissectible fat. The compartmentalization of facial fat explains the regional variation noted in the subcutaneous plane when dissecting from the preauricular area anteriorly.
- The facial fat compartments also serve as a model for deflation, confirming the observation that facial deflation in aging is compartment-specific rather than occurring homogeneously throughout the cheek.
- Facial fat compartments exist both superficial and deep to the SMAS (▶Fig. 2.1a,b and ▶Fig. 2.2).
  - The superficial facial fat, which lies within the subcutaneous plane, is superficial to the SMAS, and it is this fat which can be manipulated in an SMAS facelift.
  - Deep fat compartments, which are situated anteriorly along the orbit, maxilla, zygoma, and pyriform aperture, lie deep to the mimetic muscles and overly the periosteum of the orbit and midface. The deep fat of the cheek is contiguous with that of the lower lid. Deep malar fat along the anterior midface provides anterior cheek volume.
  - Of note, both the superficial and deep fat compartments deflate over time, and this deflation is responsible for many of the morphologic changes seen in the aging face.

2.1 Compartmentalization of the Superficial Fat Compartments

- Superficial facial fat is separated into specific compartments by the terminal extension of the deeper retaining ligaments, which percolate through the cheek from deep to superficial to insert into the skin as retinacular cutis.

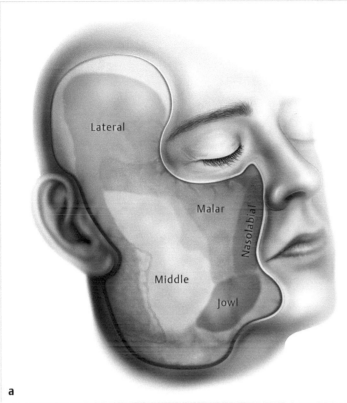
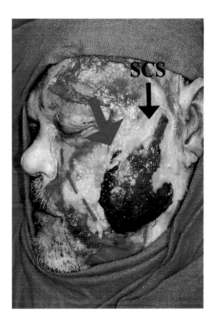

a   b

Fig. 2.1 (a) The superficial facial fat compartments are situated in the subcutaneous plane, partitioned by the terminal extensions of the retaining ligaments. The five superficial compartments of the cheek from lateral to medial are 1) lateral 2) middle 3) malar 4) jowl and 5) nasolabial. Each compartment has its own septal boundaries, a separate perforator blood supply and its own tendency to deflation in aging.
(b) Cadaver dissection of the facial fat compartments of the cheek. The inked compartment shown is the middle compartment. The red arrow marks the transition between the middle and malar compartments, which are separated by a high density of zygomatic ligaments along the lateral zygoma. (*Reproduced from Rohrich, R. Pessa, J. The Fat Compartments of the Face: Anatomy and Clinical Implications for Cosmetic Surgery. Plast. Reconstr. Surg. 119: 2219, 2007.*)

- Rather than being diffuse in their penetration of the SMAS, the retaining ligaments penetrate the superficial fascia at specific locations and thereby form the fibrous septum which are formed between compartments.
- These junctional boundaries also are the location where the vascular perforators to cheek skin penetrate from deep to superficial.
- The surgical significance of this is that when encountering numerous perforators while performing subcutaneous dissection, anatomically the dissection is transiting from one superficial fat compartment to another.
- While there are many superficial fat compartments, the five compartments that the surgeon encounters in a facelift include the lateral compartment, middle compartment, superficial malar compartment, nasolabial fold compartment, and jowl compartment.
- As subcutaneous dissection proceeds from laterally in the preauricular region medially, if the dissection is performed under direct visualization, it is possible for the physician to recognize both what compartment is being dissected as well as when the transition between compartments occurs (▶ **Fig. 2.3** and **Video 2.1**).

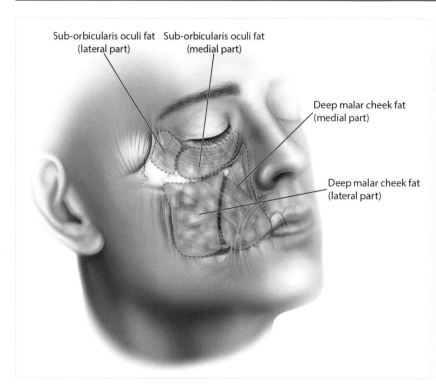

Sub-orbicularis oculi fat (lateral part)

Sub-orbicularis oculi fat (medial part)

Deep malar cheek fat (medial part)

Deep malar cheek fat (lateral part)

Fig. 2.2 The deep facial fat compartments are situated deep to the mimetic muscles and superficial to the periosteum of the midface. The deep fat of the lower lid is located just deep to the orbicularis oculi and is divided into medial and lateral components. The deep malar fat similarly is situated deep to the elevators of the upper lip and is separated into medial and lateral components. In youth, the deep periorbial fat blends with the deep malar fat to volumetrically support the lower lid and cheek. In aging, deflation of deep fat produces a loss of anterior cheek volume and an abrupt demarcation along the lid cheek junction, and it contributes to the formation of the infraorbital V-deformity.

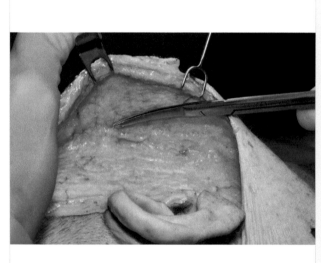

Fig. 2.3 Cadaver dissection at the junction between the middle and malar compartments along the lateral zygmoma. When transiting compartments, retaining ligaments are encountered as well as vascular perforators. The scissors in this photograph are situated where the zygomatic ligaments inset into the skin (separating the upper middle compartment from the malar compartment). The density of ligaments in this region can obscure proper plane identification, and it is safer to dissect superficially along the transition point between the middle and malar compartments, as the zygomtic motor branches lie directly sub-SMAS in this location. Notice the numerous vascular perforators present at this location, typical of vascular perforators located along transition points between compartments. Once the subcutaneous dissection proceeds anterior to the middle compartment, the mobile region of the cheek is encountered.

2.1.1 Lateral Compartment

- The lateral compartment is located in the preauricular region and tends to be narrow, thin, following the superficial temporal artery cephalically within the temporal region.

- Typically, the lateral compartment is only 3 to 5 cm in width and consists of dense, vascular, and fibrous fat.
- This compartment is directly situated overlying the parotid gland, and as the dissection proceeds anterior to the parotid, the middle compartment is encountered, and the dissection becomes less fibrous (▶ **Fig. 2.4**).

2.1.2 Middle Fat Pad

- The middle fat compartment lies medially to the parotid and lateral to the anterior boarder of the masseter.
- This compartment typically is thicker, less fibrous, and less vascular than the lateral compartment and is the compartment where most of the subcutaneous dissection of the cheek is performed in a facelift.
- Because this large compartment is thick and avascular, it tends to be easy to dissect.
- The anterior boarder of the middle compartment is bounded by the masseteric ligaments and superiorly by the zygomatic ligaments, such that the anterior boundary is adjacent to the lateral malar and jowl compartments.
- When dissecting between the middle, malar, and jowl compartments, fibrous terminal ligamentous fibers separating these compartments are encountered, and the dissection is frequently vascular, as the surgeon encounters the ascending perforators between compartments.

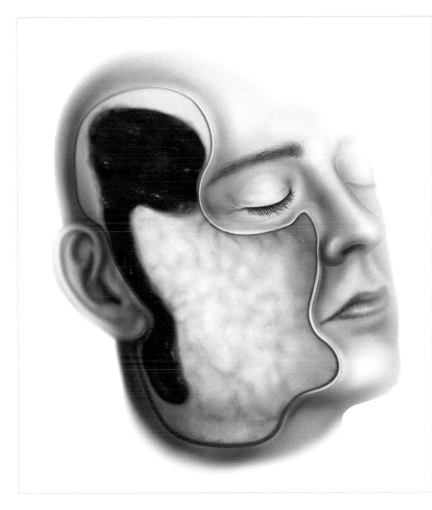

Fig. 2.4 The lateral compartment is a narrow compartment situated in the preauricular region. It overlies the parotid and superiorly extends into the temple along the path of the superficial temporal artery. The lateral compartment tends to be dense, fascial, and fibrous.

- Once the dissection proceeds anteriorly into the malar and jowl compartment, the surgeon again encounters thick, easily-dissected fat.
- The transition between the middle, malar, and jowl compartment anatomically demarcates the transition between the fixed and mobile regions of the cheek (▶ **Fig. 2.5**).

2.1.3 Superficial Malar Compartment

- The superficial malar compartment is situated along the lateral aspect of the zygomatic eminence and extends anteriorly toward the paranasal region, providing volume to the anterior cheek.
- When dissecting from the lateral cheek (middle compartment), the malar compartment is identified as the surgeon encounters numerous perforators from the transverse facial artery as well as dense fibrous zygomatic ligaments (termed McGregor's patch).
- The upper masseteric ligaments are similarly encountered along the inferior aspect of the zygoma, and the combination of dense fibrous fat with vascularity can make it difficult to accurately identify the subcutaneous plane in this region.
- As the zygomatic branches are superficially positioned just deep to the SMAS lateral to the zygoma, accurate plane identification is an important safety consideration (▶ **Fig. 2.3** and ▶ **Fig. 2.6**)

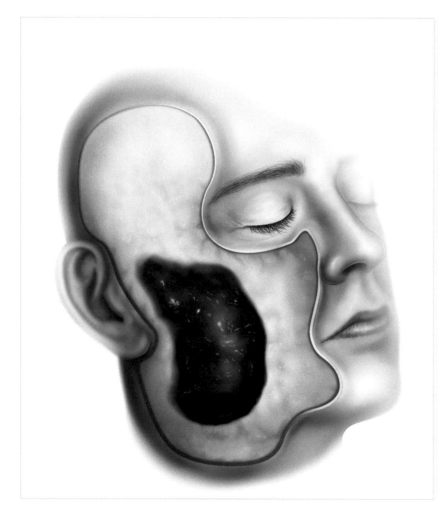

Fig. 2.5 The middle fat compartment is situated between the lateral compartment, malar, and jowl compartments. This compartment consists of thick, less vascular fat and is the compartment where most of the subcutaneous dissection is preformed in a facelift. The anterior boundary is formed by the zygomatic and masseteric ligaments, which demarcate the junction between the fixed lateral cheek and the mobile anterior cheek.

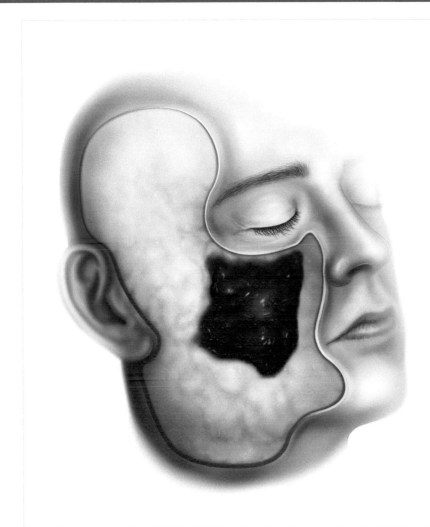

Fig. 2.6 The superficial malar fat compartment provides volume to the anterior cheek and is situated overlying the zygoma and maxilla. This compartment laterally is demarcated by the zygomatic ligaments and superiorly abuts the perioribum. This compartment of fat has also been termed the "malar fat pad" or "midface" and is the focus of many of the modern repositioning techniques for facial rejuvenation.

2.1.4 Jowl Compartment

- The jowl compartment consists of fluffy, thick fat and is situated between the mandibular ligaments and the masseteric ligaments overlying the facial portion of the platysma.
- Jowl fat tends to be avascular and easy to dissect.
- In aging, attenuation of support from the masseteric ligaments allows the platysma and overlying jowl fat to descend into the neck, which obscures the definition of the mandibular border.
- As the jowl compartment tends not to deflate in aging, jowl descent accompanied by adjacent perioral deflation is responsible for this fat compartment's becoming more apparent in middle age and elderly patients (▶ **Fig. 2.7a,b**)

2.1.5 Nasolabial Fold Compartment

- The nasolabial fold compartment sits just lateral to the nasolabial fold and anterior to the malar compartment.
- This fat compartment typically consists of thick, dense fat and rarely deflates in aging.

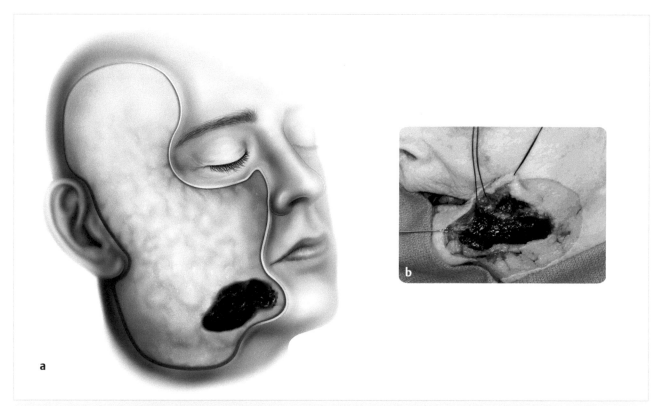

Fig. 2.7 **(a)** The jowl compartment is situated between the masseteric ligaments laterally and the mandibular ligaments medially and overlies the facial portion of the platysma. This compartment tends to consist of thick, fluffy fat and rarely deflates in aging **(b)** Cadaver dissection of jowl fat compartment. Note that the jowl fat is situated over the facial platysma, which has no deep attachement in this locaton and is supported in anatomic position by the masseteric ligaments. As this ligamentous support becomes attenuated in aging, both the platysma and jowl fat can descend into the neck, as well as radially expanding outward from the mandibular boarder, obscuring mandibular boarder definition.

- For this reason, the nasolabial compartment typically becomes more obvious in aging as the adjacent malar compartment and perioral regions deflate (▶ **Fig. 2.8**)

2.1.6 Deep Facial Fat Compartments

- The deep compartments of the cheek lie deep to mimetic muscles and overlie the periosteum of the orbit, midface, and pyriform aperture.
- The deep facial fat compartment which affects lower lid morphology is situated deep to the orbicularis oculi and is divided into a lateral and medial component.
- The anterior cheek is supported by the deep malar fat pad, which similarly has a medial and lateral component.
  - The medial component of deep malar fat is situated along the pyriform aperture and blends the perioral region with the cheek in youth.
  - The lateral component of deep malar fat contributes to anterior malar projection and blends the anterior cheek with the lateral cheek, where it abuts the buccal extension of the buccal fat pad.
  - This lateral component also abuts the orbit, blending the eyelid and cheek in youth (▶ **Fig. 2.2**).

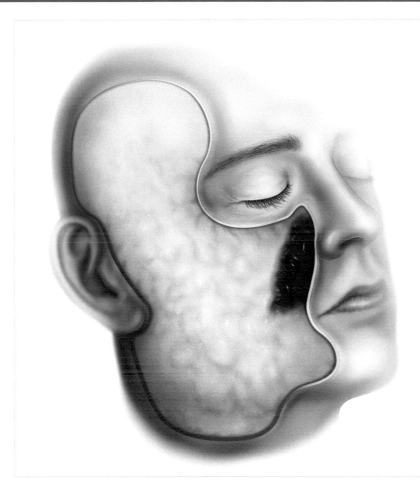

Fig. 2.8 The nasolabial compartment is situated along the pyriform aperture and is just lateral to the nasolabial fold. This compartment consists of thick, vascular fat and rarely deflates in aging.

2.2 The Anatomy of Deflation

- Facial deflation occurs with age and is responsible for many of the morphologic changes seen from youth to middle age.
- Deflation tends to be compartment-specific rather than homogeneous within the cheek, and different compartments deflate at different ages.
- Typically, early deflation of the lateral cheek becomes evident in patients in their 40s (deflation occurring within the lateral and middle compartments), while malar deflation becomes noticeable in the fifth decade.
- Malar deflation results from a loss of fat in both the superficial and deep malar compartments.
- As malar deflation affects the anterior cheek and the lower lid, the shape changes associated with malar deflation include a loss of anterior cheek volume as well as an increase in the vertical height of the lower lid (infraorbital V-deformity).
- The surgical importance of differentiating between superficial and deep deflation is that superficial deflation can be improved by repositioning superficial fat via the SMAS, while deep deflation requires volumetric augmentation for correction.
- In combination with a facelift, it is our preference to use autogenous fat grafting to correct the appearance of deep compartment deflation, adding volume in the supraperiosteal plane overlying the anterior zygoma and pyriform aperture.
- Volume addition to the deep compartment improves cheek and perioral volume as well as ameliorating the infraorbital V-deformity, shortening the vertical height of the lower lid (▶ **Fig. 2.9**).

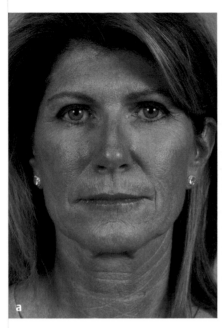 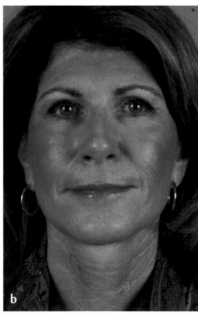

Fig. 2.9 Facial aging involves deflation of both the superficial and deep malar fat compartments. As the deep malar compartment deflates, the vertical height of the lower lid increases, the anterior cheeks lose volume, and a sharp demarcation develops between the lateral and anterior cheek where the deep malar fat abuts the buccal fat pad. This patient is seen **(a)** before and **(b)** after an extended SMAS facelift, with autologous fat grafting to the deep compartment to restore deep malar volume. (*Reproduced from Sinno, S. Mehta, K. Reavey, P. Simmons, C. Stuzin, J. Current Trends in Facial Rejuvenation: An Assessment of ASPS Members Use of Fat Grafting during Face Lifting. Plast. Recontr. Surg. 136: 20e, 2015.*)

2.3 Summary

Performing subcutaneous dissection under direct visualization with the use of transillumination to aid in precise identification of both the plane of dissection as well as the fat compartment that is being dissected increases the precision of the surgery and lessens postoperative morbidity. From a safety perspective, recognizing the transition points between compartments where facial ligaments are encountered and understanding that the relation of these transition points to facial nerve danger zones remains a key element in preventing facial nerve injury (see Chapter 3).

Suggested Readings

Gierloff M. Stohring, C. Buder, T. Gassling, V. Acil, Y. Wiltfang, J. Aging Changes of the Midface Fat Compartments: A Computed Tomographic Study. Plast Reconstr Surg. 2012; 129:263

Lambros V. Observations on periorbital and midface aging. Plast Reconstr Surg. 2007; 120(5): 1367–1376, discussion 1377

Lambros V, Stuzin JM. The cross-cheek depression: surgical cause and effect in the development of the "joker line" and its treatment. Plast Reconstr Surg. 2008; 122(5):1543–1552

Rohrich RJ, Pessa JE. The fat compartments of the face: anatomy and clinical implications for cosmetic surgery. Plast Reconstr Surg. 2007; 119(7):2219–2227, discussion 2228–2231

Rohrich RJ, Pessa JE. The retaining system of the face: histologic evaluation of the septal boundaries of the subcutaneous fat compartments. Plast Reconstr Surg. 2008; 121(5):1804–1809

Schenck T. Koban, K. Schlattau, A. Frank. K, Sykes, J. Targosinski, S. Eribacher, K/ Cptpfama, S. The Functional Anatomy of the Superfical Fat Compartments of the Face: A Detailed Imaging Study. Plast Reconstr Surg. 2018; 141:1351

Sinno S. Mehta, K, Reavey, P. Simmons, C. Stuzin, J. Current Trends in Facial Rejuvenation: An Assessment of ASPS Members Use of Fat Grafting furing Face Lifting. Plast Reconstr Surg. 2015; 136:20e

3 Overview: Facial Nerve Danger Zone

James M. Stuzin

Abstract

Facial nerve injury is a feared complication when performing facial aesthetic and reconstructive procedures. While most facial nerve branches are protected, as they are situated deep to the deep fascia as they traverse the cheek, there are specific regions of the cheek where facial nerve branches are superficially positioned and more prone to injury. These Danger Zones are located at regions of transition between facial fat compartments and are characterized by nerve branches situated in the sub-SMAS plane between superficial and deep fascia. Recognition of the plane of dissection when dissecting within Danger Zones remains a key element in preventing inadvertent motor branch injury.

Keywords: facial nerve danger zones, facial nerve injury

Key Points

- The soft tissue of the face is arranged in a series of concentric layers.
- The key point in preventing facial nerve injury is to visually recognize the plane of dissection and the relationship of this plane to the plane of the facial nerve. As long as the plane of dissection is either superficial or deep to the plane of the facial nerve, motor branch injury will be prevented.
- The thickness and visual appearance of the various facial layers will vary from patient to patient, but the concentric organization of these layers is anatomically constant (though in reoperative patients, correct plane identification can be difficult secondary to scarring).
- The position of the facial nerve in relation to these anatomic layers is similarly constant. Accurate identification of the plane of dissection (even when that layer is thin, obscure, or difficult to dissect) is the key to preventing facial nerve injury.
- In certain regions of the face, facial nerve branches penetrate the deep fascia and are situated in the plane between superficial and deep fascia before mimetic muscle innervation. Regions where these facial nerve branches are superficially positioned, in the plane between superficial and deep fascia (instead of being situated deep to the deep fascia) represent Danger Zones, as dissecting deep to the SMAS in these regions (during subcutaneous undermining) will result in motor branch injury (▶ **Fig. 3.1**).
- The facial nerve can be injured in both subcutaneous or sub-SMAS dissection. Both forms of dissection can be performed safely if the plane of the facial nerve is identified and not violated.

3.1 Safety Considerations

- The use of transillumination when dissecting the subcutaneous flap aids in accurate identification of the plane of dissection (▶ **Fig. 3.2**).
- Subcutaneous dissection is performed by definition superficial to the SMAS. If the subcutaneous anatomy is obscure and difficult to visually identify, dissecting in regions where the anatomy is easily identifiable should be performed prior to proceeding toward regions more difficult to dissect.

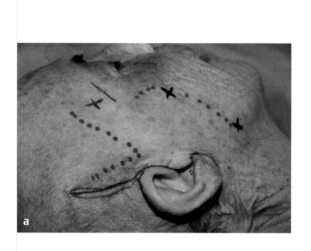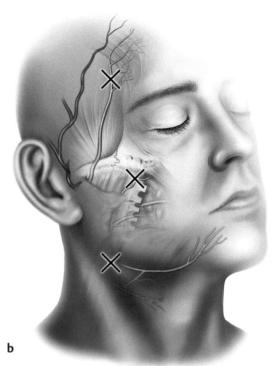

Fig. 3.1 (a) In this cadaver dissection, the areas of facial nerve Danger Zones representing the superficially situated frontal branch, zygomatic branch, and cervical branch are noted (black X). Cephalically, the red dots represent the path of the parietal and frontal branch of the superficial temporal artery. The red dots anteriorly in the cheek represent the junction between the fixed and mobile regions of the cheek demarcated by the position of the lateral zygomatic ligaments and masseteric ligaments. In terms of Danger Zones, the frontal branch is superficially positioned within the temporal region as it approaches the frontalis. The zygomatic branch is at greatest jeopardy just lateral to the zygomatic eminence where it is juxtaposed to the merging of the zygomatic and upper masseteric ligaments. The cervical branch is at greatest jeopardy along the mandibular angle, where it is juxtaposed to the caudal masseteric ligaments. Proper plane identification and inadvertent dissection deep to the SMAS should be avoided in these regions. (b) Artist illustration of the facial nerve Danger Zones of the lateral cheek. Danger Zones represent regions where facial nerve branches are superficially positioned, in the plane between the SMAS and deep fascia. Inadvertent dissection deep to the SMAS in these areas may result in motor branch injury.

- When dissecting deep to the SMAS, the sub-SMAS fat and deep facial fascia should be recognized, and the SMAS dissection kept superficial to the deep fascia. The plane of the facial nerve within the cheek lies deep to the deep fascia (▶ Fig. 3.3)

3.2 Pertinent Anatomy (Video 3.1)

3.2.1 Frontal Branch

- **After exiting the parotid,** the frontal branch overlies the periosteum of the zygomatic arch.
- Cephalad to the zygomatic arch, the frontal branch travels in the plane between the SMAS (temporoparietal fascia) and deep temporal fascia, invested in sub-SMAS fat.

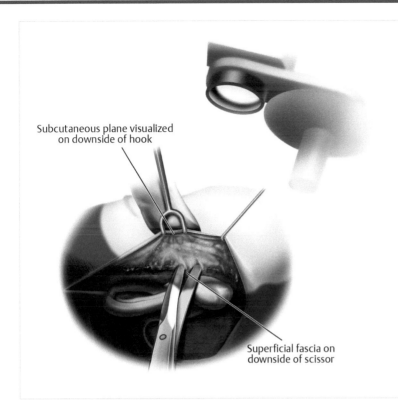

Subcutaneous plane visualized on downside of hook

Superficial fascia on downside of scissor

Fig. 3.2 Accurate plane identification is the key to safety and consistency in soft-tissue surgery of the face. The use of transillumination aids greatly in defining the interface between the subcutaneous plane and the SMAS. Performing the subcutaneous dissection under direct vision with transillumination allows greater control in terms of flap thickness and allows the surgeon to recognize the transition points between facial fat compartments, where ligaments are encountered. Recognition of these transition points, where motor branches tend to be superficially positioned, is essential in avoiding inadvertent dissection deep to the SMAS.

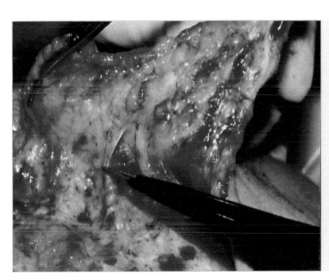

Fig. 3.3 This intraoperative photo of an extended SMAS dissection shows the elevation of the SMAS in the correct plane, superficial to the deep fascia. The hemostat in the photograph is attached to the malar portion of the dissection, while the forceps point to the upper massetertic ligaments prior to their release. Note the red fibers of the zygomaticus major are visualized medially, while laterally sub-SMAS fat is noted overlying the deep fascia. In general, it is safest to dissect in the plane between the SMAS and the sub-SMAS fat and leave the sub-SMAS fat intact along the superficial surface of the deep fascia. Nonetheless, in some patients, sub-SMAS fat is sparse, and the dissection will be adjacent to both parotid capsule and masseteric fascia (deep fascia).

- The frontal branch becomes more superficial as it traverses the temporal region and approaches the frontalis, where this mimetic muscle receives its innervation.
- As the frontal branch lies just deep to the SMAS as it approaches the frontalis, dissection deep to the SMAS in this region can produce a motor branch injury (▶ **Fig. 3.4**) (see Chapter 4).

3.2.2 Zygomatic Banch

- After exiting the parotid, the zygomatic branch lies deep to the deep fascia and overlies the masseter.
- As it approaches the zygomaticus major muscle, the zygomatic branch typically penetrates the deep fascia and becomes situated in the plane between superficial and deep fascia just inferiorlateral to the zygomatic eminence.
- In subcutaneous undermining of the cheek, the region lateral to the zygomatic eminence is both fibrous and bloody, as zygomatic ligaments, upper masseteric ligaments, and perforators from the transverse facial artery traverse this region.
- For this reason, the proper plane of dissection can be difficult to identify.
- As the zygomatic branch is superficially situated in this location, inadvertent dissection, deep to the SMAS in this location, can produce a motor branch injury resulting in upper lip weakness.
- Proper plane identification is essential in this region of the cheek, and it is often helpful to dissect the less fibrous areas of the cheek both superiorly and inferiorly to the zygomatic eminence to ensure accurate plane identification prior to dissecting in this Danger Zone (▶**Fig. 3.5**) (see Chapter 5).

3.2.3 Marginal and Cervical Branch

- The cervical branch exits the tail of the parotid and almost immediately is situated in the plane between superficial and deep fascia.
- It typically traverses the lower cheek deep to both SMAS and platysma before innervating this muscle along its deep surface.
- The cervical branch is at greatest risk of injury adjacent to the mandibular angle and caudal mesenteric ligaments.
- The caudal mesenteric ligaments tend to stout fibers and typically form a firm attachment between the skin of the lower cheek, platysma, and the underlying periosteum.
- As a result of this adherence along the angle of the mandible, the region of the caudal masseter represents a Danger Zone, as inadvertent dissection deep to the platysma will result in cervical branch injury.

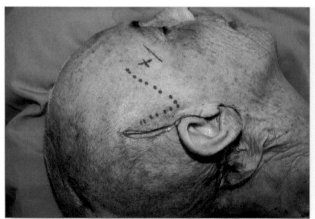

Fig. 3.4 The frontal branch is superficially positioned as it approaches the lateral frontalis in the temporal region. The area of the X marks a Danger Zone where subcutaneous dissection should be superficial and limited to prevent inadvertent motor branch injury.

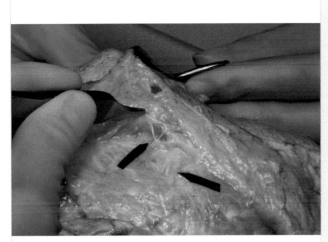

Fig. 3.5 This cadaver photograph shows both the zygomatic and buccal branches as they traverse the cheek. The lower black arrow points to the major buccal branch, which parallels the parotid duct and lies deep to the deep fascia in this location. The upper arrow points out the zygomatic branch, which innervates the zygomaticus major (held by forceps) just lateral to the zygomatic eminence. Note that this branch penetrates the deep fascia in close proximity to the transverse facial artery and lies in the plane between superficial and deep fascia in this location. As this region tends to be fibrous (zygmatic and upper masseteric ligaments) and bloody (from perforators from the transverse facial artery), plane identification can be difficult. When in doubt, dissect superficially to avoid inadvertent sub-SMAS dissection within this Danger Zone.

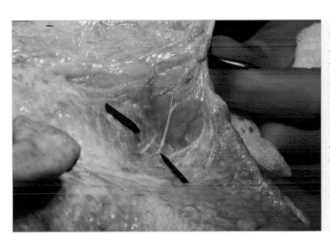

Fig. 3.6 Cadaver dissection illustrating the relationship of the marginal and cervical branches adjacent to the caudal boarder of the masseter. Note that the cervical branch (*lower arrow*) is more superficial than the marginal branch and lies just deep to the platysma (between superficial and deep fascia) before innervating this muscle. The marginal branch (*upper arrow*) lies deep to the deep fascia as it crosses the facial artery and vein, and tends to stay deep until it reaches the depressor anguli oris and inferiorus, which are innervated along their deep surfaces.

- The key to safety in subcutaneous dissection when transiting from the cheek to the neck is accurate plane identification to ensure that the dissection is carried superficial to the platysma (▶ **Fig. 3.6**).
- The marginal branch exits the tail of the parotid and is situated deep to the deep fascia, typically invested in sub-SMAS fat.
- The marginal branch remains deep to the deep fascia as it crosses the facial artery and vein and only becomes superficial when it reaches the depressors of the lower lip, which are innervated along their deep surfaces.
- Resulting from the deep position of the marginal branch as it transits across the cheek, it is infrequently injured in subcutaneous dissection.
- The marginal branch is at greater risk in sub-SMAS dissection if the dissection is carried anteriorly as far forward as the facial artery and vein (which is not necessary for adequate SMAS release).

- In this location, the caudal masseteric ligaments are dense, and the proper plane of dissection can appear obscure.
- Accurate release of the SMAS anterior to the tail of the parotid and utilizing blunt dissection once the SMAS has been freed from the parotid tail will protect the underlying marginal branch (see Chapter 6).

3.3 Technical Points

- Clearly identify and recognize the correct plane of dissection and its relation to the plane of the facial nerve (▶Fig. 3.7).
- Recognize when the dissection is proceeding adjacent to Danger Zones; only proceed to dissect in these regions after the correct plane of

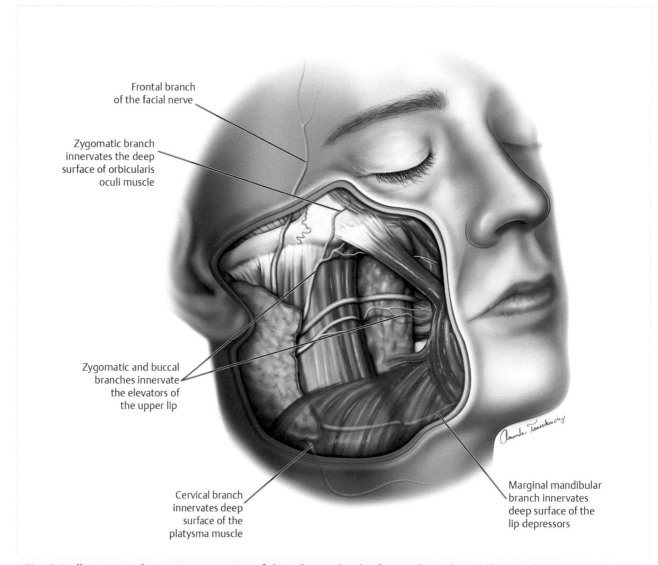

Frontal branch of the facial nerve

Zygomatic branch innervates the deep surface of orbicularis oculi muscle

Zygomatic and buccal branches innervate the elevators of the upper lip

Cervical branch innervates deep surface of the platysma muscle

Marginal mandibular branch innervates deep surface of the lip depressors

Fig. 3.7 Illustration showing an overview of the relative depth of nerve branches in the cheek. Cephalad to the zygomatic arch, the frontal branch lies in the plane between superficial and deep fascia and becomes more superficial as it travels to innervate the frontalis. The zygomatic branch is situated between the superficial and deep fascia just lateral to the zygoma, while the buccal branches typically lie deep to the deep fascia within the lateral cheek. The marginal branch lies deep to the deep fascia within the cheek, while the cervical branch is situated between superficial and deep fascia, just deep to the platysma after exiting the parotid.

dissection has been identified in areas adjacent to Danger Zones. When the dissection becomes obscure, dissect in known areas of anatomy and work back to where the anatomy is unclear. In these circumstances, PATIENCE IN PROPER PLANE IDENTIFICATION IS A KEY ELEMENT IN SAFETY.

• Recognize the appearance of the SMAS (superficial fascia) as it traverses the cheek and the visual change in its appearance as it transits between facial fat compartments.

• When elevating SMAS flaps in the cheek, recognize the appearance of both the parotid capsule and masseteric fascia and dissect superficial to these layers. Leaving sub-SMAS fat intact overlying the deep fascia and dissecting directly along the undersurface of the SMAS provides an extra layer of protection between SMAS elevation and the more deeply situated facial nerve branches.

Suggested Readings

Alghoul M, Bitik O, McBride J, Zins JE. Relationship of the zygomatic facial nerve to the retaining ligaments of the face: the Sub-SMAS danger zone. Plast Reconstr Surg. 2013; 131(2): 245e–252e

Baker DC, Conley J. Avoiding facial nerve injuries in rhytidectomy. Anatomical variations and pitfalls. Plast Reconstr Surg. 1979; 64(6):781–795

Dingman RO, Grabb WC. Surgical anatomy of the mandibular ramus of the facial nerve based on the dissection of 100 facial halves. Plast Reconstr Surg Transplant Bull. 1962; 29:266–272

Freilinger G, Gruber H, Happak W, Pechmann U. Surgical anatomy of the mimic muscle system and the facial nerve: importance for reconstructive and aesthetic surgery. Plast Reconstr Surg. 1987; 80(5):686–690

Furnas DW. The retaining ligaments of the cheek. Plast Reconstr Surg. 1989; 83(1):11–16

Pitanguy I, Ramos AS. The frontal branch of the facial nerve: the importance of its variations in face lifting. Plast Reconstr Surg. 1966; 38(4):352–356

Roostaeian J, Rohrich RJ, Stuzin JM. Anatomical considerations to prevent facial nerve injury. Plast Reconstr Surg. 2015; 135(5):1318–1327

Seckel B. Facial Nerve Danger Zones. 2nd ed. Boca Raton, Fl.: CRC Press; 2010

Stuzin JM, Wagstrom L, Kawamoto HK, Wolfe SA. Anatomy of the frontal branch of the facial nerve: the significance of the temporal fat pad. Plast Reconstr Surg. 1989; 83(2):265–271

Tzafetta K, Terzis JK. Essays on the facial nerve: Part I. Microanatomy. Plast Reconstr Surg. 2010; 125(3):879–889

4 Frontal Branch of the Facial Nerve

James M. Stuzin

Abstract

Differing from other facial nerve branches, after exiting the parotid, the frontal branch lies in the plane between superficial and deep fascia. Safe dissection within the temporal region should therefore be carried either superficial or deep to the plane of the frontal branch, as sub-SMAS dissection in the temporal region may result in motor branch injury. A knowledge of deep temporal fascia anatomy and its relation to the temporal fat pad is useful in preventing motor branch injury in procedures requiring subperiosteal dissection of the zygomatic arch.

Keywords: frontal branch anatomy, frontal branch injuries

Key Points

- After exiting the parotid and traveling cephalad to the zygomatic arch, the frontal branch penetrates the deep fascia and is situated in the plane between superficial and deep fascia as it traverses the temporal region towards the frontalis.
- The soft tissue layers of the temporal region are a bit different than the layers of the lower cheek. These layers include the skin, subcutaneous fat, the SMAS (also termed temporparietal fascia), the loose areolar layer (also termed subaponeurotic fascia) which contains sub-SMAS fat, and the deep fascia (also termed deep temporal fascia).
- From patient to patient, the soft tissue of the temporal region exhibits a variable degree of thickness, but the anatomic concentric relationship of these layers is constant. The frontal branch within the temporal region is situated within the loose areolar supaponeurotic plane (between superficial and deep fascia) invested in the sub-SMAS fat. This motor branch tends to become more superficial (lying just deep to the SMAS), where it innervates the frontalis along the lateral orbital rim. The region just lateral to the superior orbital rim therefore represents a Danger Zone if the subcutaneous dissection is carried deep to the SMAS (►**Fig. 4.1**).
- Two-dimensionally, there is variability in terms of frontal nerve branching patterns, and this nerve can exist as a single branch or multiple (up to six) branches as it travels within the temporal region. Pitanguy's line, marking the general path of the frontal branch within the temporal region, is a useful guide for the general path of the frontal nerves and is along a tangent drawn between the base of the tragus and a landmark 1.5 cm above the eyebrow (►**Fig. 4.2**).
- Despite variations in branching patterns, all frontal motor branches are situated anterior and inferior to the frontal branch of the superficial temporal artery. For this reason, the frontal branch of the superficial temporal artery is a key landmark when dissecting within the temporal region (►**Fig. 4.3a,b**).

- In terms of Danger Zones within the temporal region, inadvertent dissection deep to the superficial fascia (SMAS) can injure the underlying frontal branches of the facial nerve. For this reason, dissection of the temporal region must be performed superficial to the SMAS in the subcutaneous plane during a facelift dissection.
- In procedures such as browlifting or craniofacial procedures requiring exposure of the zygomatic arch, dissection should be carried either directly overlying the deep temporal fascia or just deep to the superficial layer of the deep temporal fascia within the superficial temporal fat pad. This deep dissection in the temporal region will protect superficially situated motor branches (▶Fig. 4.4).
- The key to safety remains accurate identification of the plane of dissection and understanding the depth of the plane of dissection in relation to the plane of the frontal branch (▶Fig. 4.5).

4.1 Safety Considerations

- Use of transillumination when dissecting the subcutaneous flap aids in accurate identification of the subcutaneous plane of dissection.
- The temporal region tends to be thin, with a paucity of subcutaneous fat overlying the superficial fascia. Ensuring that the dissection is kept superficial to the SMAS is the key to preventing inadvertent deep dissection.
- Ligating the parietal branch of the superficial temporal artery in performing the "meso-temporalis" temporal dissection when performing a facelift is safe, as the parietal branch of the artery is posterior to the path of the motor branches. If the anterior (frontal) branch of the superficial temporal artery is encountered, the surgeon should be cognizant that this is an important landmark, and the motor branches are situated just anterior and inferior to this structure (▶Fig. 4.3).

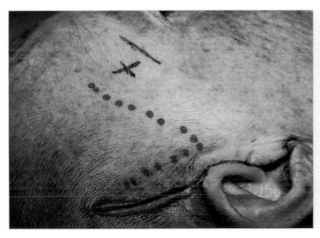

Fig. 4.1 After exiting the parotid, the frontal branch traverses the temporal region in the plane between superficial and deep fascia invested in sub-SMAS fat. This nerve branch tends to become more superficial as it travels toward the lateral boarder of the frontalis juxtaposed to the lateral orbital rim. Inadvertent dissection deep to the SMAS in this region (X) therefore represents a Danger Zone, and the surgeon should insure dissection remains superficial to the SMAS. The dotted red lines represent the paths of the parietal and frontal branches of superficial temporal artery. Frontal nerve branches are always situated caudal to the frontal branch of the superficial temporal artery.

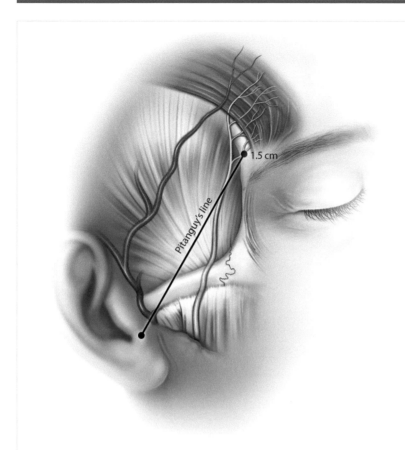

Fig. 4.2 Pitanguy's line is the classic reference line for the general path of the frontal branch within the temporal regions. This landmark is a line from the base of the tragus to 1.5 cm above the eyebrow. While Pitanguy's line is a useful reference, the frontal branches can be situated in any location between the frontal branch of the superficial temporal artery and Pitanguy's line (though these branches three-dimensionally are always situated between superficial and deep fascia).

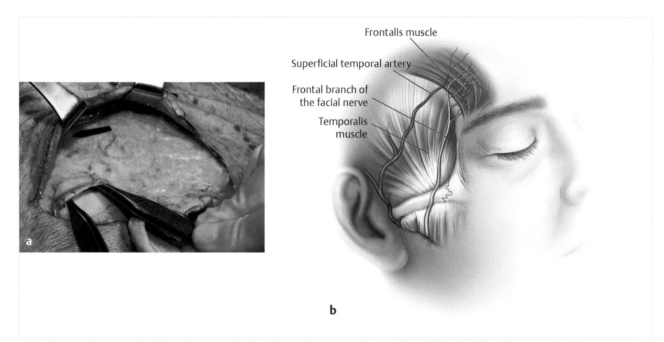

Fig. 4.3 **(a)** The superficial temporal artery has two main branches, a parietal branch shown in this cadaver dissection and a frontal branch, which is situated anteriorly and lies invested within the SMAS (*black arrow*). Motor nerve branches are always situated anterior to the frontal branch of the superficial temporal artery. Notice the thickness of the SMAS of the temporal region, which invests these arterial branches. Note also the thickness of the soft tissue of the temporal region between the subcutaneous plane and the deep temporal fascia. It is this soft tissue which not only invests the arterial branches but more deeply also invests the frontal nerve motor branches.
(b) Illustration of the frontal nerve branch and its relationship to the frontal branch of the superficial temporal artery.

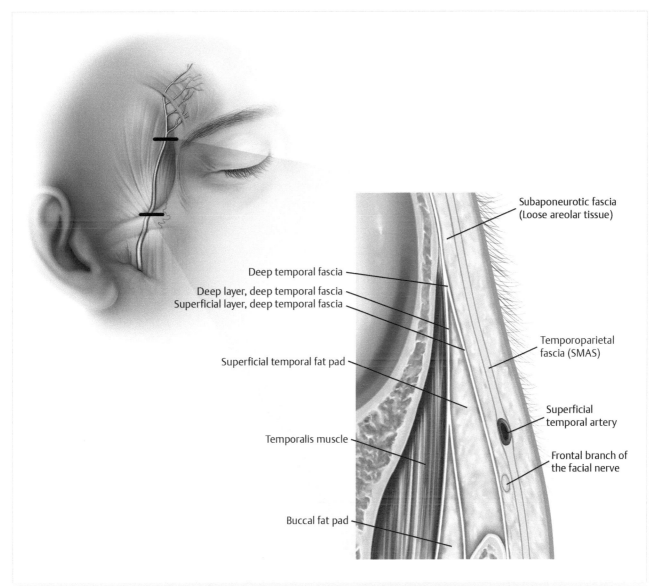

Deep temporal fascia

Deep layer, deep temporal fascia

Superficial layer, deep temporal fascia

Superficial temporal fat pad

Temporalis muscle

Buccal fat pad

Subaponeurotic fascia
(Loose areolar tissue)

Temporoparietal
fascia (SMAS)

Superficial
temporal artery

Frontal branch of
the facial nerve

Fig. 4.4 A cross section of the temporal region illustrated in the region between the superior orbital rim and the zygomatic arch. The superficial fascia (SMAS) invests the superficial temporal artery, while deep to the SMAS (in the plane between superficial and deep fascia) is the loose areolar layer, termed subaponeurotic fascia, which contains sub-SMAS fat. The frontal nerve branches are situated in the subaponeurotic plane invested in the sub-SMAS fat. The deep temporal fascia splints into two layers caudal to the superior orbital rim to encase the superficial temporal fat pad. In craniofacial procedures requiring exposure of the zygomatic arch, it is preferable to dissect deep to the superficial layer of the deep temporal fascia, within the superficial temporal fat pad, rather than directly superficial to the deep temporal fascia, as this will provide greater protection again motor branch injury.

4.2 Danger Zones and Clinical Correlation-Pertinent Anatomy (Video 4.1)

- After exiting the parotid, the frontal branch directly overlies the periostium of the zygomatic arch.
- Cephalad to the zygomatic arch, the frontal branch travels in the plane between the SMAS (temporal parietal fascia) and deep temporal fascia, invested in sub-SMAS fat.

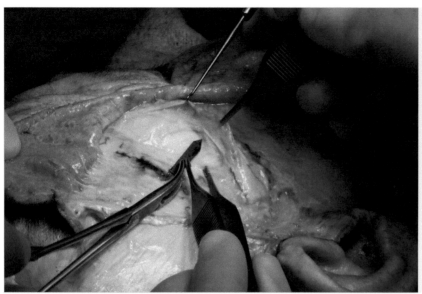

Fig. 4.5 A cadaver dissection demonstrating the frontal branch within the temporal region (*arrow*). The frontal branch lies within the loose areolar layer (also termed subaponeurotic fascia) invested in sub-SMAS fat. This plane is just deep to the SMAS and is superficial to the deep temporal fascia. The key to safety when operating in the temporal region is to dissect either superficial or deep to the plane of the frontal branch.

- The frontal branch becomes more superficial as it traverses the temporal region and approaches the frontalis. This mimetic muscle, similar to most mimetic muscles, is innervated along its deep surface.
- As the frontal branch lies just deep to the SMAS, inadvertent dissection deep to the SMAS within the temporal region can produce a motor branch injury (▶ **Fig. 4.6** and ▶ **Fig. 4.7**).
- The general path of the frontal branch is on a line from the base of the tragus to a landmark 1.5 cm cephalad to the eyebrow.
- When performing an extended SMAS dissection, keeping the cephalad limit of the dissection caudal to the general path line of the frontal branch is an important safety consideration (see chapter 8).
- As emphasized, as the frontal branch lies in the plane between superficial and fascia within the entire temporal region, inadvertent deep dissection beneath the SMAS can produce a motor branch injury. Subcutaneous dissection superficial to the SMAS is safe, and transillumination to define the plane between subcutaneous fat and the SMAS is helpful when dissecting in this region.
- Alternatively, when performing dissection in the temporal region such as required in browlifting or in exposure of the craniofacial skeleton and zygomatic arch, dissection deep to the frontal branch is preferred.
- For these procedures, dissecting along the superficial surface of the deep temporal fascia is safe until the superior orbital rim is encountered.
- Caudal to the superior orbital rim, it is preferable to incise the superificial layer of the deep temporal fascia and continue the dissection within the superficial temporal fat compartment toward the zygomatic arch. Dissecting deep to the deep temporal fascia in this region provides another layer of protection against injuring the more superficially situated motor branches.
- Another safety consideration is to recognize the thickness of the subaponeurotic facia (loose areolar layer), which is situated between the SMAS and the deep temporal fascia.
  - This loose areolar layer marks the plane of the frontal branch, and the sub-SMAS fat visible in this layer is the structure that invests the motor branches within the temporal region.

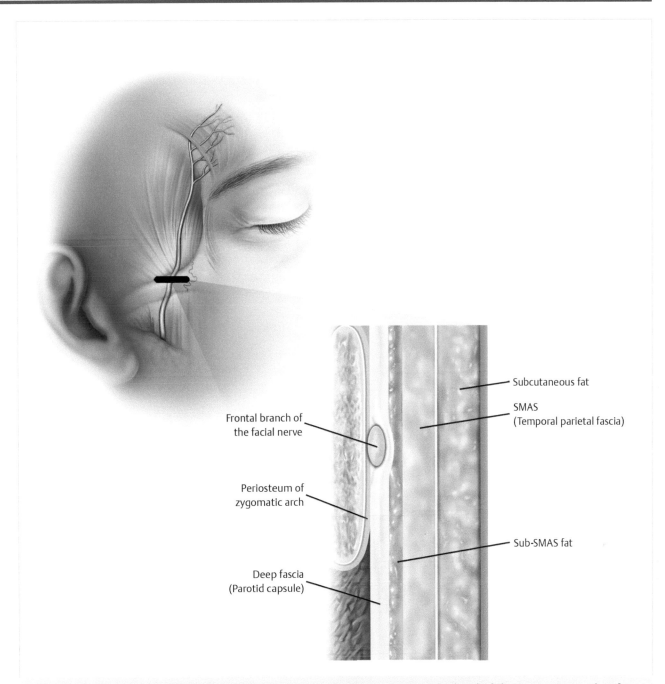

Fig. 4.6 A cross section of the frontal branch after it exits the parotid, at the level of the zygomatic arch. After exiting the parotid, the frontal branch directly overlies the periostium of the zygomatic arch. Cephlad to this location, the frontal branch penetrates the deep fascia and becomes situated in the plane between the SMAS and the deep termporal fascia (between superficial and deep fascia) as it traverses the temporal region.

– When performing browlifting-type procedures, dissect just superficial to the deep temporal fascia, and keep the subaponeurotic fascia attached to the forehead flap. As the orbital rim is approached, sub-SMAS fat becomes evident, and this fat (which marks the plane of the frontal branch) should be recognized and the dissection carried deep to this layer (▶ Fig. 4.7).

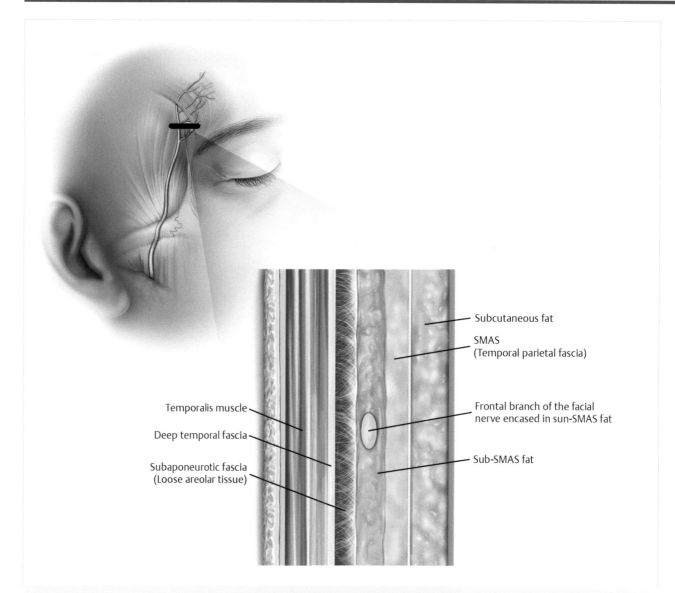

Fig. 4.7 A cross section of the frontal branch at the level of the superior orbital rim, prior to innvervating the frontalis. At this level, the frontal branch lies just deep to the SMAS (temporoparietal fascia) encased in sub-SMAS fat and juxtaposed to the loose areolar subaponuerotic fascia. When dissecting within the temporal region in procedures such as browlifting, it is important to dissect along the superficial surface of the deep temporal fascia and leave the loose areolar layer intact up on the scalp flap to protect the more superficially positioned frontal branch. A KEY POINT TO REMEMBER IS THAT THE LOOSE AREOLAR LAYER WITHIN THE TEMPLE IS ALSO THE PLANE OF THE FRONTAL BRANCH.

4.3 Technical Points

- Clearly identify the plane of dissection, and recognize its relation to the plane of the frontal branch when dissecting in the temporal region.
- When performing a cervicofacial flap either for a face lift or reconstructive procedures, the preferred plane of dissection in the temporal region is in the subcutaneous plane superficial to the SMAS.
- When performing a browlift or in dissections requiring exposure of the craniofacial skeleton and zygomatic arch, the safe plane of dissection

within the temporal region is the plane between the deep temporal fascia and the loose areolar subaponeurotic fascia.
- Caudal to the level of the superior orbital rim, the deep temporal fascia splits to encase the superficial temporal fat pad. When dissecting in the temporal region caudal to the superior orbital rim, the preferred dissection plane is to incise the superficial layer of the deep temporal fascia and dissect toward the zygomatic arch deep to the superficial layer of the deep temporal fascia, within the superficial temporal fat pad.

Suggested Readings

Moss CJ, Mendelson BC, Taylor GI. Surgical anatomy of the ligamentous attachments in the temple and periorbital regions. Plast Reconstr Surg. 2000; 105(4):1475–1490, discussion 1491–1498

Pitanguy I, Ramos AS. The frontal branch of the facial nerve: the importance of its variations in face lifting. Plast Reconstr Surg. 1966; 38(4):352–356

Roostaeian J, Rohrich RJ, Stuzin JM. Anatomical considerations to prevent facial nerve injury. Plast Reconstr Surg. 2015; 135(5):1318–1327

Seckel B. Facial Nerve Danger Zones. 2nd ed. Boca Raton, Fl.: CRC Press; 2010

Stuzin JM, Wagstrom L, Kawamoto HK, Wolfe SA. Anatomy of the frontal branch of the facial nerve: the significance of the temporal fat pad. Plast Reconstr Surg. 1989; 83(2):265–271

Tzafetta K, Terzis JK. Essays on the facial nerve: Part I. Microanatomy. Plast Reconstr Surg. 2010; 125(3):879–889

Trussler AP., Stephan P, Hatef D, et al. The Frontal Branch of the Facial Nerve across the Zygomatic arch: anatomical relevance of the high-SMAS

5 Zygomatic and Buccal Branches

James M. Stuzin

Abstract

The zygomatic and buccal branches lie deep to the deep fascia after exiting the parotid. While protected in this location, a branch to the zygomaticus major penetrates the deep fascia to lie within the sub-smas plane just lateral to the zygomatic eminence, representing a Danger Zone for inadvertent deep dissection. Buccal branches tend to become more superficially positioned as they traverse anteriorly in the cheek overlying the buccal fat pad, and dissection deep to the deep fascia in this region may result in motor branch injury.

Keywords: zygomatic and buccal branch anatomy, zygomatic and buccal branch injury

Key Points

- The zygomatic and buccal branches of the facial nerve lie deep to the deep facial fascia after exiting the parotid. Typically, there are multiple variations in terms of branching patterns and numerous interconnections between these particular motor branches.
- The zygomatic branches and buccal branches are responsible for innervation to the elevators of the lip. The zygomatic branches also innervate the orbicularis oculi as well as provide innervation to the glabella musculature.
- After exiting the parotid, both the zygomatic and buccal branches are situated deep to the deep fascia overlying the masseter and penetrate the deep fascia anteriorly when they reach the mimetic muscles which they innervate. As previously noted, most mimetic muscles are innervated along their deep surfaces (▶Fig. 5.1 and ▶Fig. 5.2).
- The zygomatic motor branch to the zygomaticus major is an exception in terms of the plane it traverses within the cheek. This branch typically penetrates the deep fascia lateral to the zygomatic eminence and just lateral to the zygomaticus major, situated in the plane between superficial and deep fascia. For this reason, the region just inferior and lateral to the zygomatic eminence represents a danger zone, and dissection deep to the SMAS in this location may produce inadvertent motor branch injury, resulting in upper lip weakness (▶Fig. 5.3 and ▶Fig. 5.4a,b)
- Anatomically, lateral to the zygomatic eminence, a high density of retaining ligaments is located, formed by a merging of both the zygomatic and upper mesenteric ligaments. Subcutaneous dissection in this region is typically fibrous as these ligamentous fibers are encountered.
- In subcutaneous dissection, the region just lateral of the zygomatic eminence represents a transition zone between the middle and malar fat compartments. This region is not only fibrous but also vascular as perforators from the transverse facial artery are encountered. In some patients, this may result in difficulty in terms of accurately identifying the subcutaneous plane. THE KEY TO SAFETY IS ACCURATE PLANE IDENTIFICATION: THE DISSECTION IN THIS LOCATION SHOULD BE CARRIED SUPERFICIAL TO THE SMAS TO PREVENT MOTOR BRANCH INJURY (▶Fig. 5.5).

• Buccal branches of the facial nerve are always situated deep to the deep fascia, though they become more superficial as they course anteriorly. A major zygomatic/buccal branch typically parallels the parotid duct, though this branch is deep and infrequently injured. The more superficially positioned buccal branches, noted anterior and inferior in the cheek overlying the buccal fat pad, may be injured if the dissection is carried deep to both the SMAS and deep fascia. Thin patients with little subcutaneous and sub-SMAS fat or reoperative patients are at greater risk for inadvertent deep dissection and buccal branch injury (▶Fig. 5.2).

5.1 Safety Considerations

• The use of transillumination when dissecting the subcutaneous flap aids in accurate identification of the proper plane of dissection.
• Subcutaneous dissection should be performed superficial to the SMAS. The subcutaneous anatomy can become obscure and difficult to visually identify when encountering retaining ligaments along the lateral zygomatic eminence and along the anterior boarder of the masseter, when transiting facial fat compartments.
• The region where the ligaments are at highest density is along the lateral zygomatic eminence where the zygomatic and upper mesenteric ligaments are situated. As the zygomatic branch is superficial in this location, accurate plane identification and superficial dissection will prevent a motor branch injury.
• Buccal branch injury is most likely when encountering ligaments along the anterior boarder of the masseter. Accurate plane identification when encountering these ligaments and ensuring the dissection remains superficial to the SMAS will prevent a motor branch injury.

5.2 Danger Zones and Clinical Correlation-Pertinent Anatomy (Video 5.1)

• It can be difficult from an anatomic perspective to differentiate zygomatic from buccal branches.
• These nerve branches both participate in upper lip elevation and in smiling.

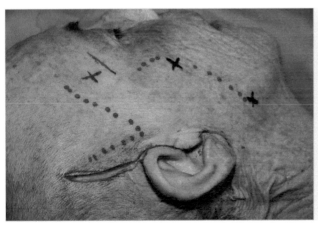

Fig. 5.1 After exiting the parotid, the zygomatic branch overlies the masseter and lies deep to the deep fascia within the midcheek. This nerve branch tends to become more superficial as it travels to the zygomaticus major and typically penetrates the deep fascia just lateral to the zygoma.

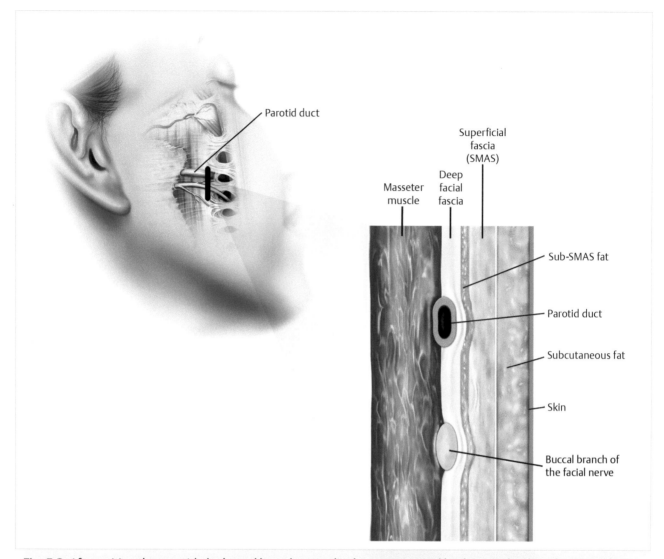

Fig. 5.2 After exiting the parotid, the buccal branches overlie the masseter and lie deep to the deep fascia. As the mimetic muscles innervated by the buccal branches are situated medially, buccal branches remain deep to the deep fascia as they traverse superficial to the buccal fat pad and then penetrate the deep fascia when reaching the muscles innervated. A large zygomatic/buccal branch parallels the parotid duct deep to the deep fascia within the midcheek.

- The superior branches are termed zygomatic branches, and the lower branches are termed buccal branches.
- Once exiting the parotid, these nerve branches overlie the masseter and are situated deep to the deep facial fascia (▶ Fig. 5.1 and ▶ Fig. 5.2).
- The zygomatic branch to the zygomaticus major typically penetrates the deep fascia just lateral to the zygomatic eminence and is situated in the plane between superficial and deep fascia in this location.
- The region lateral to the zygomatic eminence, is both fibrous and vascular, making plane identification difficult in some patients in a location where motor branches are superficially positioned (▶ Fig. 5.3, ▶ Fig. 5.4, ▶ Fig. 5.5).
- The buccal branches lie more caudal to the zygomatic branches, and a major buccal branch parallels the parotid duct.

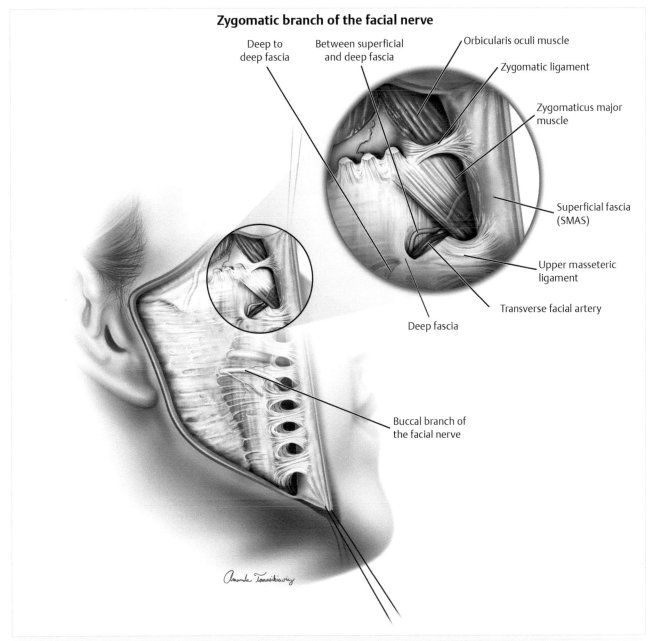

Zygomatic branch of the facial nerve

Deep to deep fascia

Between superficial and deep fascia

Orbicularis oculi muscle

Zygomatic ligament

Zygomaticus major muscle

Superficial fascia (SMAS)

Upper masseteric ligament

Transverse facial artery

Deep fascia

Buccal branch of the facial nerve

Fig. 5.3 The region directly lateral to the zygomatic eminence (middle X) is a danger zone for potential injury to the zygomatic branch, which innervates the zygomaticus major. Typically, the zygomatic branch is superficially positioned in this location, in the plane between superficial and deep fascia. This location also exhibits high ligamentous density, as the zygomatic and upper masseteric ligaments merge in this region.

- The inferior buccal branches become more superficial as they traverse the cheek. Along the anterior border of the masseter, the masseteric ligaments bind the skin and the superficial and deep fascia to the masseter.
- The masseteric ligaments of the midcheek (mid-masseteric ligaments) typically are fine, thin fibers, such that plane identification is usually straight forward. Nonetheless, inadvertent deep dissection in this region, which represents the transition between the middle, malar, and jowl compartments, may result in buccal branch injury (▶ **Fig. 5.6**).

43

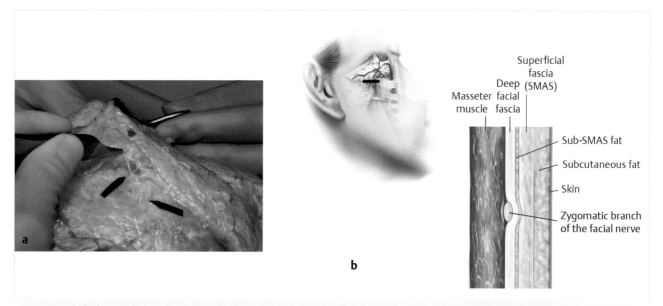

Fig. 5.4 **(a)** This cadaver photograph illustrates the superficial position of the zygomatic branch in the region just lateral to the zygomatic eminence. In this photograph, the SMAS has been reflected to delineate the sub-SMAS plane. The forceps retract the zygomaticus major. The zygomatic branch in this location is situated in the plane between the superficial and deep fascia, crossing the transverse facial artery to innervate the zygomaticus major along its deep surface (*upper arrow*). The lower arrow points to the parotid duct and the major buccal branch which parallels the parotid duct. Both of these structures are situated deep to the deep fascia in the midcheeek. **(b)** Artist illustration of the above photograph demonstrating the sub-SMAS plane lateral to the zygomatic eminence. Note that the zygomatic branch lies directly sub-SMAS (in the plane between superficial and deep fascia) in this location, while the parotid duct and buccal branches are more deeply situated, deep to the deep fascia.

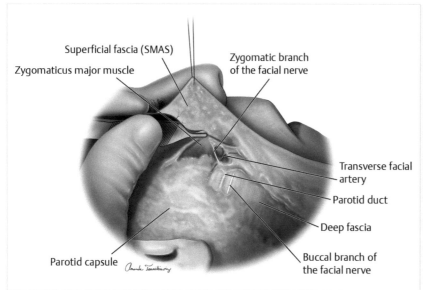

Fig. 5.5 Illustration demonstrating the penetration of the deep fascia by the zygomatic branch just lateral to the malar eminence. Note that this superficially positioned branch is juxtaposed to both the transverse facial artery as well as fibers from the zygomatic and upper masseteric ligaments. The combination of a superficially positioned motor branch in a region that is both vascular and fibrous mandates accurate plane identification as this danger zone is dissected.

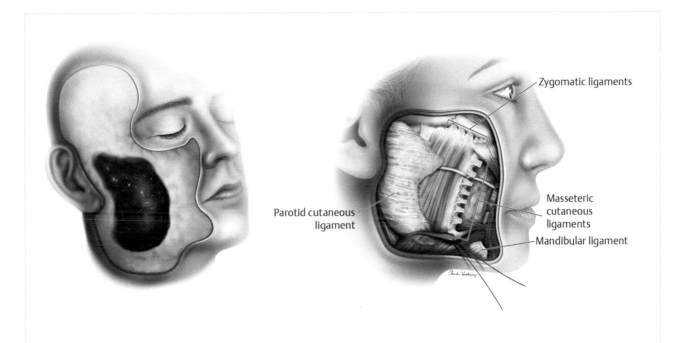

Fig. 5.6 (a,b) The masseteric ligaments separate the middle fat compartment from the malar and jowl compartments. When transiting compartments from the lateral to medial cheek, both ligaments and vascular perforators will be encountered. In this location, the buccal branches remain situated deep to the deep fascia. Nonetheless, in thin patients with little subcutaneous or sub-SMAS fat or in reoperative situations, accurate plane identification may prove difficult, leading to inadvertent deep dissection and buccal branch injury. RECOGNIZE WHEN THE DISSECTION TRANSITS COMPARTMENTS AND ENSURE THE DISSECTION REMAINS SUPERFICIAL TO THE SMAS.

5.3 Technical Points

- Clearly identify the correct plane of dissection and its relation to the plane of the facial nerve. In subcutaneous undermining, the correct plane of dissection is superficial to the SMAS. In sub-SMAS dissection, the correct plane of dissection is superficial to the deep fascia.
- Recognize when the dissection is adjacent to Danger Zones.
- The Danger Zone for the zygomatic branch is in the region of the lateral zygomatic eminence. Dissection in this region will be fibrous and vascular, as the zygomatic and mesenteric ligaments are encountered as well as perforators of the transverse facial artery. If the dissection becomes obscure, it is safest to dissect in known areas of anatomy, both cephalad and caudal to this region, to ensure dissection is carried superficial to the SMAS as this Danger Zone is approached.
- When dissecting in the midcheek along the anterior border of the masseter, the fibers of the mid-masseteric ligaments will be encountered along the transition between the middle, malar, and jowl fat compartments. This ligamentous adherence can similarly make identification of the proper plane of dissection difficult. Performing dissection superficial to the SMAS will prevent inadvertent motor branch injury.

- In performing an extended SMAS dissection, the superficial fascia (SMAS) is dissected from the parotid, accessory lobe of the parotid and the superior aspect of the zygomaticus major muscle.
  - The key to safety in sub-SMAS dissection is to identify the parotid capsule and deep fascia and not to dissect deep to this fascial layer.
  - In terms of safety, we find it helpful to dissect just along the deep surface of the SMAS and leave the underlying sub-SMAS fat undisturbed overlying the deep fascia. Leaving the sub-SMAS fat intact serves as a layer of protection between the SMAS dissection and the underlying facial nerve branches (see Chapter 8).

Suggested Readings

Alghoul M, Bitik O, McBride J, Zins JE. Relationship of the zygomatic facial nerve to the retaining ligaments of the face: the Sub-SMAS danger zone. Plast Reconstr Surg. 2013; 131(2):245e–252e

Baker DC, Conley J. Avoiding facial nerve injuries in rhytidectomy. Anatomical variations and pitfalls. Plast Reconstr Surg. 1979; 64(6):781–795

Mendelson BC, Muzaffar AR, Adams WP, Jr. Surgical anatomy of the midcheek and malar mounds. Plast Reconstr Surg. 2002; 110(3):885–896, discussion 897–911

Mendelson BC, Jacobson SR. Surgical anatomy of the midcheek: facial layers, spaces, and the midcheek segments. Clin Plast Surg. 2008; 35(3):395–404, discussion 393

Roostaeian J, Rohrich RJ, Stuzin JM. Anatomical considerations to prevent facial nerve injury. Plast Reconstr Surg. 2015; 135(5):1318–1327

Seckel B. Facial Nerve Danger Zones. 2nd ed. Boca Raton, FL: CRC Press; 2010

Skoog T. Plastic Surgery- New Methods and Refinements. Philadelphia: WB Saunders; 1974

Stuzin JM, Baker TJ, Gordon HL. The relationship of the superficial and deep facial fascias: relevance to rhytidectomy and aging. Plast Reconstr Surg. 1992; 89(3):441–449, discussion 450–451

Tzafetta K, Terzis JK. Essays on the facial nerve: Part I. Microanatomy. Plast Reconstr Surg. 2010; 125(3):879–889

6 Protecting the Marginal and Cervical Branches of the Facial Nerve

James M. Stuzin

Abstract

The marginal and cervical branches function to coordinate lower lip movement and lower lip depressor function. The marginal branch innervates the depressor anguli oris, inferioris, mentalis, and orbicularis oris, while the cervical branch innervates the platysma. There are many interconnections between nerve branches, coordinating animation. While the marginal branch is deeply positioned deep to the deep fascia, the cervical branch is more superficially positioned in the sub-SMAS plane, such that dissection deep to the platysma may result in motor branch injury. The Danger Zone for cervical branch injury is located at the transition between the middle and jowl fat compartments, adjacent to the caudal masseteric ligaments separating these compartments.

Keywords: danger zones, marginal and cervical branch, facial nerve injury

Key Points

- The two-dimensional branching patterns of the marginal and cervical branches of facial nerve are variable, making it difficult to ascertain exact nerve location when dissecting within the cheek and neck.
- On a three-dimensional basis, the position and depth of the marginal and cervical branches are constant and predictable.
- Understanding the three-dimensional anatomy in terms of planes of dissection, as well as the Danger Zones where these nerve branches are vulnerable to injury, provides protection against iatrogenic injury when preforming surgical rejuvenation of the aging face.
- The greatest risk of cervical branch injury is along the mandibular boarder adjacent to the caudal extent of the masseteric ligaments, in the region of the angle of the mandible.
- When dissecting from the cheek toward the cervical region, ensure the dissection is subcutaneous and stays superficial to the platysma.

6.1 Safety Considerations

- Both the marginal and cervical branches lie deep to the superficial fascia (SMAS) and platysma.
- Subcutaneous dissection superficial to the SMAS and platysma is safe. Accurate identification of the SMAS and platysma defines the subcutaneous plane.
- The cervical branch is more superficial than the marginal and is therefore more frequently injured.
- The cervical branch is at greatest risk as it innervates the platysma along the mandibular angle, adjacent to the caudal masseteric ligaments.
- As the caudal masseteric ligaments extend from the masseter through the platysma into the overlying skin, encountering these fibers when

dissecting from the cheek toward to the cervical region can obscure proper plane identification. As the cervical branch is superficially positioned in this location, inadvertent dissection deep to the platysma may result in motor branch injury.

- The cervical branches may also be injured in sub-SMAS dissection where the nerve penetrates the deep fascia anterior to the tail of the parotid. Blunt dissection in this region during SMAS elevation is helpful in preventing nerve injury.

- The intramuscular cervical branches within the platysma may be injured during defatting of the neck by inadvertent dissection into the platysma muscle. These types of injuries are usually transient and heal quickly. Injury to a major cervical branch often requires 4 to 8 weeks to recover.

- The marginal branch is situated deeply, deep to the deep fascia within the cheek, and is infrequently injured.

6.2 Pertinent Anatomy (Video 6.1)

- The marginal and cervical branches of the facial nerve are interconnected in both an anatomic and functional relationship, working together in lower lip animation. Cross-nerve connections between the cervical and marginal branches are frequently noted in cadaver dissection, attesting to how these two nerve branches communicate to coordinate lower lip function (▶ Fig. 6.1).

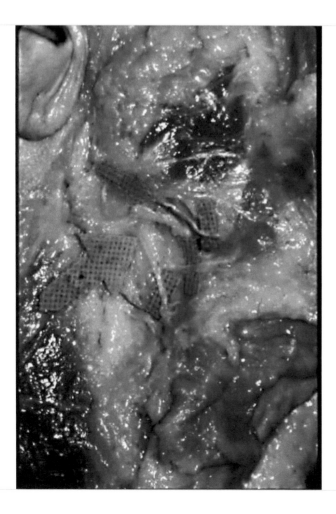

Fig. 6.1 This cadaver photograph illustrates the interconnections between the marginal and cervical branches. The large arrow points to the cervical branch, while the smaller arrow marks the more deeply situated marginal branch. An interconnection between these branches is commonly noted as these nerves communicate function during animation.

- In general, the cervical branch is the dominate innervation for the platysma, while the marginal branch provides the dominate innervation for the depressor anguli oris, depressor inferioris, mentalis, and orbicularis oris.
- The key to safety when preforming both subcutaneous or sub-SMAS/ platysma dissection within the cheek and neck is to accurately understand the depth of these nerve branches as they traverse the cheek and neck.
- DEPTH OF THE MARGINAL BRANCH: After exiting anterior to the tail of the parotid, the marginal branch lies deep to the deep fascia encased in sub-SMAS fat. Even in emaciated cadavers, the presence of sub-SMAS fat overlying the marginal branch just anterior to the tail of the parotid is visible and serves as a valuable landmark for nerve location.
- As it travels toward the lower lip, the marginal branch lies deep to the deep fascia and is tightly bound by the deep fascia to the masseter and mandible as it crosses superficial to the facial artery and vein (▶ **Fig. 6.2**).
- Coursing peripherally toward the lower lip, the marginal branch lies deep to the deep fascia until it reaches the depressors of the lower lip. In this location (beginning with the Depressor Anguli Oris) the marginal branch penetrates the deep fascia and innervates the lower lip depressors along their deep surface. Some branches course deeply toward the mentalis, which, unlike most mimetic muscles, is innervated along its superficial surface (▶ **Fig. 6.3**).
- DEPTH OF THE CERVICAL BRANCH: There tends to be significant variability in the number and location of cervical branches. After exiting anterior to the tail of the parotid, the cervical branch penetrates the deep fascia and travels within the sub-SMAS plane, situated between the deep surface of the platysma and the underlying deep facial fascia.
- Even when traveling adjacent to the marginal branch, because the cervical nerve traverses within the sub-SMAS plane, this branch lies superficial to the marginal nerve and is therefore at greater risk for iatrogenic injury if dissection is carried inadvertently deep to the platysma. This anatomic fact accounts for the frequency of cervical branch injury as compared to the rarity of marginal branch injury (▶ **Fig. 6.4a,b** and ▶ **Fig. 6.5**).

6.3 Danger Zones and Clinical Correlations

6.3.1 Cervical Branch

- Topographically, the caudal boarder of the masseter marks a Danger Zone for inadvertent cervical branch injury. The anatomic rationale for this is that the caudal masseteric ligaments tend to be substantive and thereby tightly bind the skin and platysma to the underlying deep fascia and masseter in this region, adjacent to the jawline and mandibular boarder (▶ **Fig. 6.6**).
- The cervical branch is at greatest risk for injury in thin patients with little paucity of subcutaneous fat.
  - The Danger Zone for nerve injury which is defined by the caudal masseteric ligaments is encountered when dissecting from the cheek inferiorly toward the neck along the mandibular boarder. Because of the density of the ligaments in this location, it can be difficult to identify the proper plane of dissection.

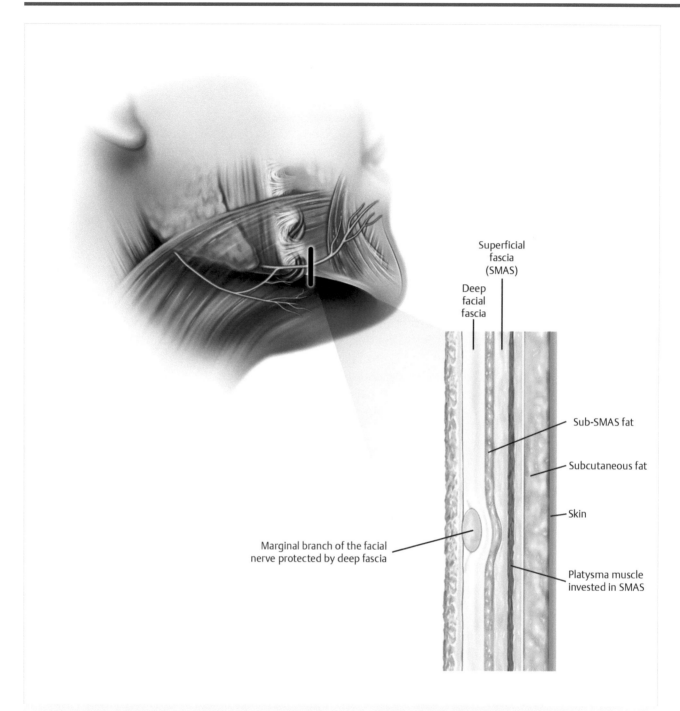

Superficial
fascia
(SMAS)

Deep
facial
fascia

Sub-SMAS fat

Subcutaneous fat

Skin

Marginal branch of the facial
nerve protected by deep fascia

Platysma muscle
invested in SMAS

Fig. 6.2 The marginal branch is illustrated in a cross section taken just anterior to the facial artery and vein along the mandibular boarder. In this location, it is situated deep to the deep fascia. It remains in this relatively protected deep position until it reaches the depressor anguli oris and depressor inferiorus, which are innervated along their deep surfaces.

- You can feel this region of "Danger Zone" on your own jawline. Clinch your teeth and place your index finger along the caudal aspect of the anterior boarder of the masseter. Pick up the skin along the anterior boarder, and when you pinch the skin inferiorly along the jawline and mandible, notice how the skin is fixed and much less mobile than more superiorly in the cheek. This adherence demonstrates the most caudal fibers of the masseteric ligaments and can make subcutaneous dissection difficult between skin and platysma.

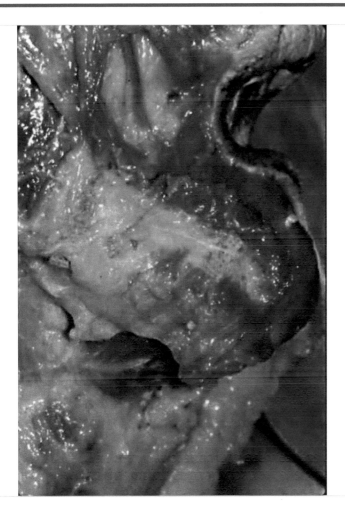

Fig. 6.3 This cadaver photograph traces the marginal branch deep to the depressor anguli oris and depressor inferiorus. As demonstrated, these muscles are innervated along their deep surfaces.

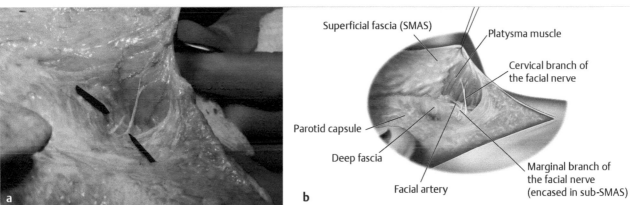

Superficial fascia (SMAS)

Platysma muscle

Cervical branch of the facial nerve

Parotid capsule

Deep fascia

Facial artery

Marginal branch of the facial nerve (encased in sub-SMAS)

a

b

Fig. 6.4 (a) Cadaver dissection demonstrating the cervical branch (situated in the plane between superficial and deep fascia) and its relation to the marginal branch and facial artery and vein, which lie deep to the deep fascia along the angle of the mandible (upper arrow). The lower arrow points to where the cervical branch innervates the platysma (*forceps*). Dissection deep to the platysma in this location may result in motor branch injury. **(b)** Artist's illustration demonstrating the superficial position of the cervical branch, situated between the superficial and deep fascia along the angle of the mandible. The marginal branch, facial artery and vein lie deep to the deep fascia in this location.

- The cervical branch typically enters the deep surface of the platysma at this point in many patients, such that if the dissection is carried through the platysma in this "zone," an injury to the cervical branch is likely.

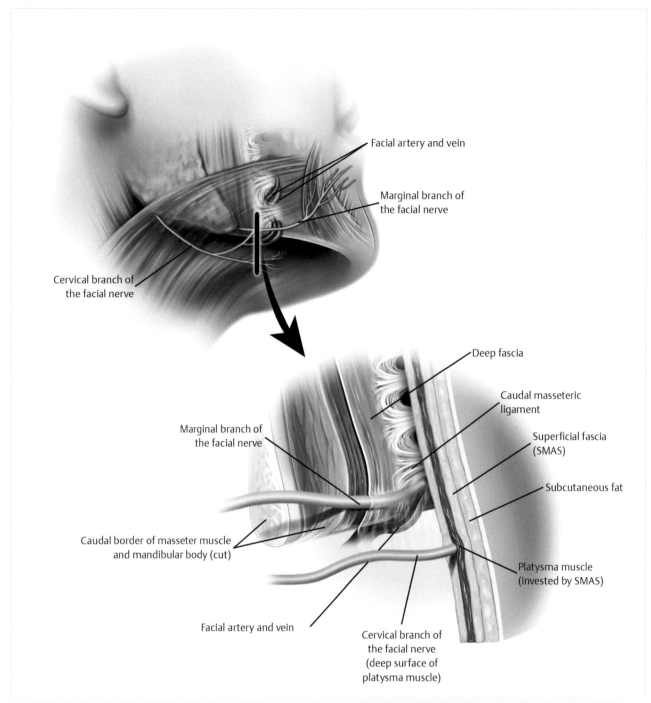

Fig. 6.5 Cross section illustrating the relative depths of the marginal and cervical branches along the angle of the mandible. Note the proximity of the caudal masseteric ligaments, which bind the skin to the caudal masseter in this location. The deeply situated marginal branch is relatively protected in this location, while the superficially positioned cervical branch is in greater jeopardy from inadvertent deep dissection.

- Fortunately, the marginal branch is bound to the mandible and masseter by the deep fascia in this location and is thereby protected.
- In terms of nerve recovery, the marginal nerve is dominant for lower-lip depressor function, such that full recovery is typically noted 4 to 8 weeks following cervical branch injury.

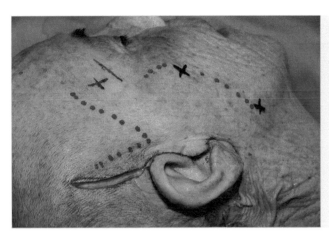

Fig. 6.6 The lower X marks the Danger Zone for injury to the cervical branch. Note that this region is demarcated by the caudal masseteric ligaments and angle of the mandible. The cervical branch typically is situated directly deep to the platysma in this location, in the plane between superficial and deep fascia.

- The cervical branch can also be injured when preforming SMAS flap elevation or platysma window procedures. The key to safety is careful SMAS dissection overlying the parotid and anterior SCM. As the SMAS flap is elevated anteriorly, accurate identification of the cervical nerve branches is essential, followed by blunt dissection in the areolar plane anterior to the parotid and SCM to avoid branch injury.

6.3.2 Marginal Branch

- The marginal branch is infrequently injured in either subcutaneous or sub-SMAS dissection because of its deep location. In either subcutaneous or sub-SMAS dissection, as long as the plane of the deep fascia is not violated, marginal branch injury will be prevented.
- In terms of safety in sub-SMAS dissection/platysma window techniques, after the SMAS is released from the retaining ligaments along the tail of the parotid and anterior boarder of the SCM, an areolar plane is encountered anteriorly between superficial and deep fascia.
- As the dissection is carried anterior to the tail of the parotid, the sub-SMAS fat lying deep to the deep fascia and marking the location of the marginal branch is easily identified.
- In most patients, the marginal branch is not apparent in sub-SMAS dissection, as it remains covered by this sub-SMAS fat. As previously noted, the key to prevention of nerve injury is to NOT violate the deep fascia during surgical undermining.
- After identifying the loose areolar layer anterior to the parotid and SCM, gentle blunt dissection between the superficial and deep fascia will protect both the marginal and cervical branches while allowing adequate release of the SMAS/platysma flap.

6.4 Summary

As with other facial nerve branches, the key to avoiding motor branch injury is accurate identification of the plane of dissection and understanding its relation to the plane of the facial nerve. The cervical branch is the most commonly injured branch in facelifting procedures, resulting from the anatomic fact that after it exits the parotid, cervical branches are situated in the plane between superficial and deep fascia, just deep to the platysma. Inadvertent dissection deep to the platysma should be avoided during subcutaneous dissection. After these branches enter the deep surface of the platysma they travel intramuscularly such that dissection into the muscle anteriorly (especially along the region of the mandibular boarder) can also produce temporary lower lip weakness. This most commonly occurs during submental cervical dissection and defatting. Fortunately, the marginal branch is dominant, and this paresis is temporary. When defatting the neck, the key to safety is to recognize the superficial surface of the platysma and leave the fascia overlying this muscle intact.

Suggested Readings

Baker DC, Conley J. Avoiding facial nerve injuries in rhytidectomy. Anatomical variations and pitfalls. Plast Reconstr Surg. 1979; 64(6):781–795

Dingman RO, Grabb WC. Surgical anatomy of the mandibular ramus of the facial nerve based on the dissection of 100 facial halves. Plast Reconstr Surg Transplant Bull. 1962; 29:266–272

Freilinger G, Gruber H, Happak W, Pechmann U. Surgical anatomy of the mimic muscle system and the facial nerve: importance for reconstructive and aesthetic surgery. Plast Reconstr Surg. 1987; 80(5):686–690

Roostaeian J, Rohrich RJ, Stuzin JM. Anatomical considerations to prevent facial nerve injury. Plast Reconstr Surg. 2015; 135(5):1318–1327

Seckel B. Facial Nerve Danger Zones. 2nd ed. Boca Raton, FL: CRC Press; 2010

Stuzin JM, Baker TJ, Gordon HL. The relationship of the superficial and deep facial fascias: relevance to rhytidectomy and aging. Plast Reconstr Surg. 1992; 89(3):441–449, discussion 450–451

Tzafetta K, Terzis JK. Essays on the facial nerve: Part I. Microanatomy. Plast Reconstr Surg. 2010; 125(3):879–889

7 Great Auricular Nerve

James M. Stuzin

Abstract

The great auricular nerve is a sensory branch innervating the earlobe and lateral cheek. It is perhaps the most commonly injured nerve when performing a facelift. The key to inadvertent injury is a three-dimensional understanding of the relationship of this nerve to the superficial cervical fascia and SCM as it traverses the lateral neck. This chapter discusses great auricular nerve anatomy and emphasizes methods to avoid inadvertent injury.

Keywords: danger zone great auricular nerve, great auricular nerve injury

Key Points

- The great auricular nerve is a sensory branch derived from the cervical plexus, receiving its innervation from C2 and C3. The great auricular nerve provides sensation to the skin of the preparotid region, the lower ear, and ear lobe.
- Injury to the great auricular nerve results in numbness of these regions and in some cases neuroma formation, resulting in painful dysethesia.
- The great auricular nerve is always situated lateral to the external jugular vein, a useful landmark as this vein is often visible externally (▶ Fig. 7.1).
- The classical location for identifying the nerve is described as McKinney's Point, located along the middle of the sternocleidomastoid muscle 6.5 cm inferior to the external auditory canal (▶ Fig. 7.2).
- In terms of depth, the great auricular nerve is situated deep to the cervical fascia overlying the SCM and lateral platysma. The cervical fascia overlying the SCM is in continuity with the SMAS of the cheek (▶ Fig. 7.3).
- Subcutaneous dissection superficial to the cervical fascia overlying the SCM will prevent inadvertent injury to the great auricular nerve.

7.1 Safety Considerations

- When dissecting in the postauricular region, recognize the fascia overlying the sternocleidomastoid muscle, and do not dissect deep to this fascial layer.
- If the fibers of the sternocleidomastoid muscle are exposed during dissection, recognize that the plane of dissection is inadvertently deep.
- The great auricular nerve is at greatest jeopardy during postauricular dissection as the undermining is carried along the posterior boarder of the SCM. In this region, the cervical skin is typically adherent to the SCM, and in many patients, subcutaneous fat is sparse in this location, making plane identification difficult.
- Significant differences in branching patterns of the great auricular nerve exist from patient to patient. Typically, there is a posterior and anterior branch as well as a branch to the earlobe. These branches become more superficial as they enter the earlobe and are frequently visible in this location.

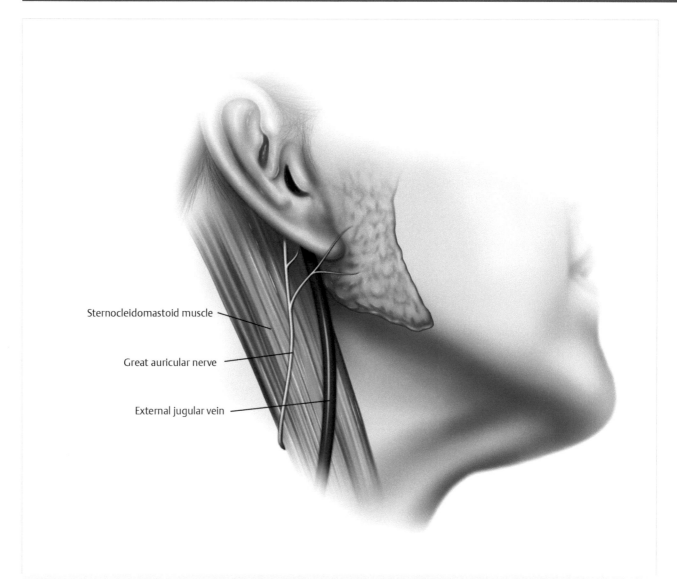

Fig. 7.1 The great auricular nerve is a branch of the cervical plexus providing sensory innervation to the earlobe and lateral cheek. It typically consists of an anterior and posterior branch as well as a branch to the earlobe. The great auricular nerve is situated lateral to the external jugular vein.

- While McKinney's point is a useful landmark to identify the path for the great auricular nerve, we have noted patient variability in terms of the relationship of this nerve to the middle of the SCM. In some patients, especially in patients with a vertically long neck, the great auricular nerve will cross the middle of the SCM low in the neck and then become situated along the anterior border of the sternocleidomastoid muscle. In this anterior location, the great auricular nerve is at risk during sub-SMAS dissection and platysma window techniques (▸ **Fig. 7.4**).

7.2 Danger Zones and Clinical Correlation-Pertinent Anatomy

- After exiting Erb's point along the posterior border of the sternocleido-mastoid muscle, the great auricular nerve travels across the SCM toward the ear.

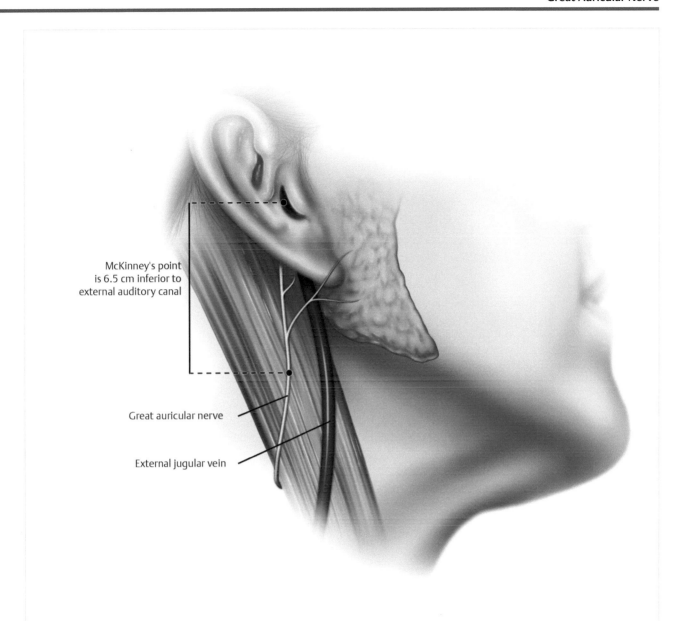

McKinney's point
is 6.5 cm inferior to
external auditory canal

Great auricular nerve

External jugular vein

Fig. 7.2 McKinney's point is a classic reference point for the great auricular nerve. It is a point 6.5 cm inferior to the external auditory canal and demarcates where the great auricular nerve crosses the middle of the SCM. While it is a useful landmark, the great auricular nerve can be injured at any point if the dissection is inadvertently carried deep to the cervical fascia.

- Most patients exhibit a posterior and anterior branch as well as a branch to the earlobe lobule. These branches become more superficial as they ascend in the neck; it is not uncommon during dissection adjacent to the lobule to encounter nerve branches.
- While it is classically taught that the great auricular nerve crosses the midbelly of the SCM 6.5 cm below the auditory canal, there is some degree of patient variability as to the location of the nerve in relation to the SCM. Nonetheless, in all patients this nerve branch is situated deep to the SMAS/platysma and cervical fascia overlying the SCM.
- The key to safety when operating in the postauricular region is to recognize the cervical fascia overlying the anterior surface of the

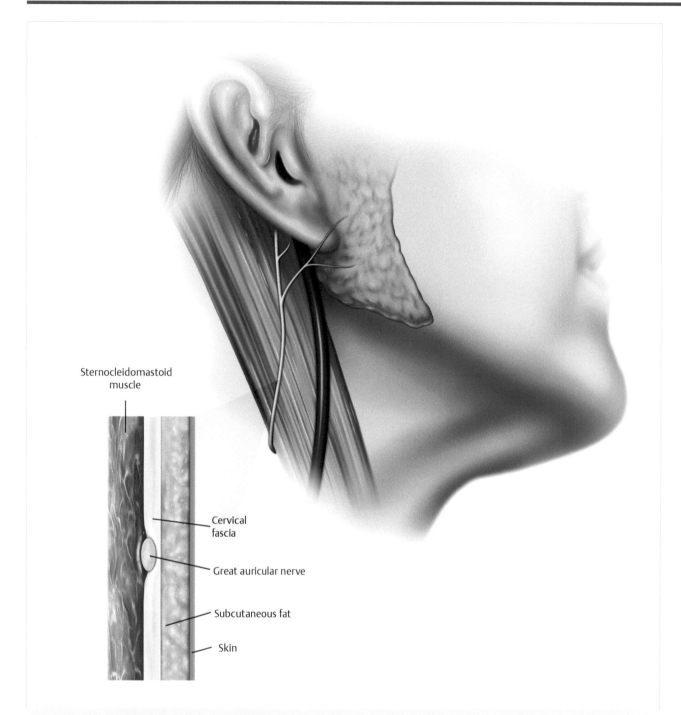

Sternocleidomastoid
muscle

Cervical
fascia

Great auricular nerve

Subcutaneous fat

Skin

Fig. 7.3 The key to preventing injury to the great auricular nerve is an accurate understanding of the depth of dissection in relation to the depth of the nerve. Despite variations in branching patterns, the great auricular nerve is always situated deep to the cervical fascia overlying the SCM. As long as the dissection is kept superficial to the cervical fascia, nerve injury will be prevented.

sternocleidomastoid and perform the subcutaneous underming superficial to this layer. As the great auricular nerve is always situated deep to the cervical fascia, if the muscle fibers of the SCM become evident during dissection, recognize that the plane of dissection is inadvertently deep (▶ **Fig. 7.3**).

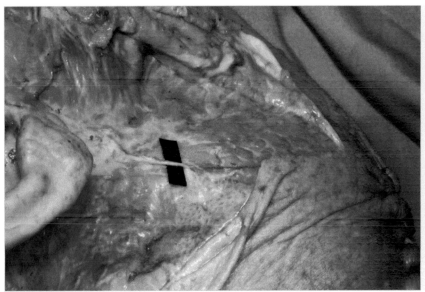

Fig. 7.4 Photograph demonstrating the path of the great auricular nerve, situated in this cadaver overlying the SCM. While McKinney's point is the classic reference point for the path of this sensory branch, there are variations in terms of the vertical trajectory of this nerve and its relation to the SCM. Three-dimensional anatomy is constant, and the great auricular nerve is always situated deep to both the cervical fascia overlying the SCM and the platysma.

7.3 Technical Points

- As dissection in the postauricular region is frequently fibrous and vascular, it is important to recognize the correct plane of dissection, which is the subcutaneous plane superficial to the cervical fascia overlying the sternocleidomastoid muscle.
- In terms of safety, recognize when the cervical fascia has been violated, exposing the fibers of the sternocleidomastoid muscle. If the muscle is visible, realize that the dissection in inadvertently deep, and ensure that further dissection is superficial to the fascia. It is helpful to utilize transillumination to identify the subcutaneous plane.
- The area of greatest jeopardy for nerve injury is when dissecting in the lower neck along the posterior boarder of the SCM. As the ligamentous adherence in this region is dense and there is typically sparse subcutaneous fat, care is required to dissect superficial to the cervical fascia at this location. Using blunt dissection if the plane of dissection is unclear is useful in nerve protection.
- While McKinney's point is a useful landmark, there is variability as to where the great auricular nerve crosses the SCM. The key to safety is not McKinney's point but rather recognizing the depth of dissection. As the great auricular nerve always is situated deep to the cervical fascia, dissection in the subcutaneous plane superficial to the fascia will prevent nerve injury.
- When performing a lateral platysma window technique or in sub-SMAS dissection along the lateral platysma border, it is important to realize that the great auricular nerve can be in close proximity. A technical point to prevent nerve injury is that after incising the lateral platysma, dissect directly along the undersurface of the platysma, and ensure that the plane of dissection avoids anteriorly positioned nerve branches. Blunt dissection is useful after the lateral platysma has been incised (**Video 7.1**).

Suggested Readings

McKinney P, Katrana DJ. Prevention of injury to the great auricular nerve during rhytidectomy. Plast Reconstr Surg. 1980; 66(5):675–679

Seckel B. Facial Nerve Danger Zones. 2nd ed. Boca Raton, FL: CRC Press; 2010

Baker TJ, Gordon HL, Stuzin JM. Surgical Rejuvenation of the Face. 2nd ed. St Louis, Mosby Year-Book; 1996

Stuzin JM. MOC-PSSM CME article: Face lifting. Plast Reconstr Surg. 2008; 121(1, Suppl):1–19

8 Technical Considerations: Extended SMAS Dissection and Lateral SMASectomy/Platysma Window

James M. Stuzin

Abstract

The basis for modern facelift techniques is to utilize the SMAS to reposition facial fat from the anterior cheek into regions of lateral cheek and malar deflation, restoring the volumetric highlights noted in youth. This chapter discusses two commonly utilized techniques: the Extended SMAS Dissection and Lateral SMASectomy/Platysma Window, emphasizing both technique and methods to avoid inadvertent motor branch injury when performing a facelift.

Keywords: extended and high SMAS technique, lateral SMAS ectomy and SMAS stacking technique, platysma window technique

---

Key Points: Extended SMAS Dissection

- If an extended SMAS dissection is planned (sub-SMAS dissection of the lateral cheek superficial fascia in continuity with the malar fat pad), the key to successfully performing this procedure is precise subcutaneous dissection.
  - Leaving substantial subcutaneous fat intact along the superficial surface of the SMAS will provide a thick SMAS flap, which is technically easier to dissect.
  - Transillumination is helpful in accurate skin flap dissection (▶Fig. 8.1).
- When beginning the SMAS dissection, identifying the plane between the SMAS and the underlying parotid capsule is important. As dissection proceeds anteriorly, an essential point is to not violate either the parotid capsule or deep fascia during sub-SMAS dissection. This protects against parotid fistula and motor nerve injury.
- Sub-SMAS fat is apparent after the SMAS has been elevated anteriorly from the lateral parotid capsule. Leaving the sub-SMAS fat intact along the superficial surface of the deep fascia, dissecting in the interface between the undersurface of the SMAS and the sub-SMAS fat, provides greater protection against injuring motor branches situated deep to the deep fascia (▶Fig. 8.2a,b).
- The limits of sub-SMAS dissection are reached when transiting from the fixed to mobile regions of the SMAS, past the restraint of the retaining ligaments.
- Typically, the extent of SMAS dissection requires freeing the superficial fascia from the parotid, lateral zygoma, upper masseteric ligaments, and the anterior board of the SCM (▶Fig. 8.3).

8.1 Safety Considerations

- Most of an extended SMAS dissection overlies areas where the facial nerve is protected. The majority of SMAS elevation occurs overlying the

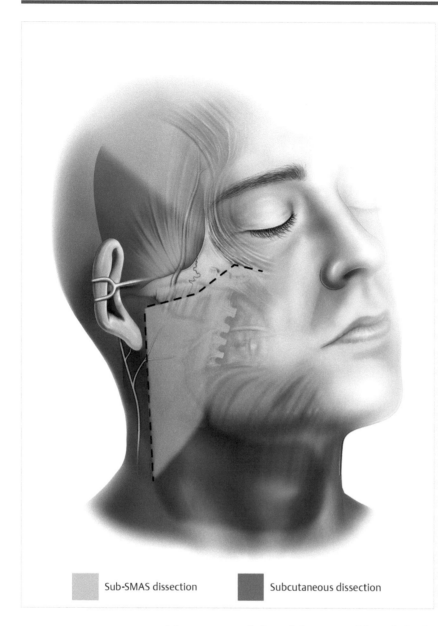

Fig. 8.1 The incision for an extended SMAS dissection is shown in this illustration. The limits of sub-SMAS dissection required to release the SMAS from fixed structures are also noted. This incision design allows release of the SMAS of the lateral cheek and malar pad from the restraint of the retaining ligaments and provides the opportunity to reposition anterior facial fat into regions of deflation in the upper lateral cheek, restoring the volumetric highlights noted in youth.

Sub-SMAS dissection   Subcutaneous dissection

parotid, accessory lobe of the parotid and the lateral zygoma, all regions where facial nerve branches are protected.

- The regions where the nerve branches are in jeopardy lie anterior to the parotid and along the region lateral to the zygomatic eminence.
- Once the SMAS is dissected from its attachments to the parotid, lateral zygoma, and upper masseteric ligaments, the dissection can has reached the mobile region of the SMAS. At this point, the dissection is less fibrous as it has proceeded past the restraint of the retaining ligaments.
  - ONCE THE DISSECTION BECOMES EASY, STOP, as the SMAS flap is released and further dissection produces little additional movement in terms of repositioning facial fat.
- Limiting the dissection within the mobile region of the SMAS minimizes the risk to motor nerve injury, which are more exposed in the anterior region of the cheek.
- Directly lateral to the zygoma, the SMAS requiring dissection tends to become thin as it transits from the lateral cheek superiorly along the superficial surface of the zygomaticus major. The upper masseteric

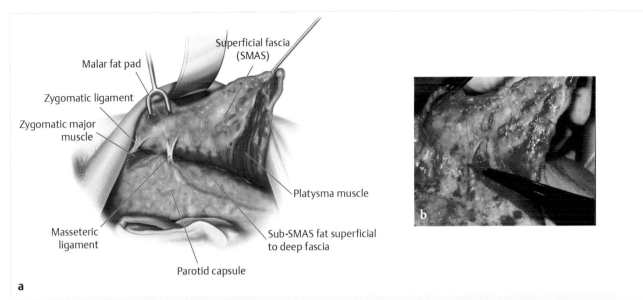

Superficial fascia
(SMAS)

Malar fat pad

Zygomatic ligament

Zygomatic major
muscle

Masseteric
ligament

Platysma muscle

Sub-SMAS fat superficial
to deep fascia

Parotid capsule

a

b

Fig. 8.2 (a) The key to sub-SMAS dissection is accurate identification of the plane between superficial and deep fascia. As the parotid capsule represents deep fascia, keeping the dissection superficial to this layer is a key element following initial incision in an extended SMAS dissection. Anterior to the parotid, the deep (masseteric) fascia is encountered. It is our preference to keep the sub-SMAS fat intact along the superficial surface of the deep fascia, as this adds an extra layer of protection against inadvertent deep dissection. (b) Intraoperative photos of an Extended Smas dissection. The hemostat is placed on the malar fat pad along the lateral zygoma, exposing the zygomaticus major. The forceps are pointing to the upper masseteric ligament, which requires release to access the mobile sub-SMAS region of the lateral cheek.

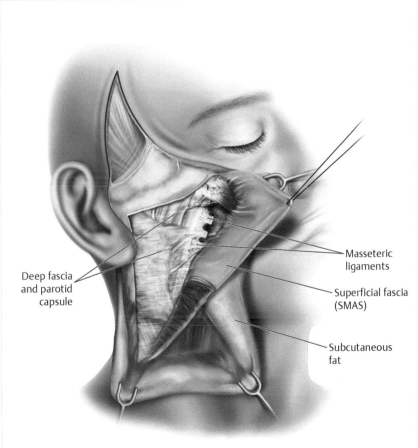

Deep fascia
and parotid
capsule

Masseteric
ligaments

Superficial fascia
(SMAS)

Subcutaneous
fat

Fig. 8.3 The limits of an extended SMAS dissection are reached when the SMAS is freed from the anterior boarder of the parotid, the accessory lobe of the parotid, the lateral zygomatic ligaments, the upper masseteric ligaments, and the anterior boarder of the SCM. Once the sub-SMAS dissection is freed from these structures and the dissection carried into the mobile sub-SMAS region of the lateral cheek, further dissection is unnecessary in terms of the release required to reposition facial fat. Of note, the incision and dissection required in the platysma window technique is analogous to the lateral/inferior dissection of the platysma illustrated in this diagram.

ligaments are encountered in this region as well as the transverse facial artery. Care in accurate plane identification is essential in this region of the dissection, for both motor branch protection as well as to not tear the SMAS flap as it is dissected from the upper masseteric ligaments (►**Fig. 8.2b**).

- Once the SMAS is dissected from the upper masseteric ligaments, the mobile region of the smas is encountered. The dissection becomes less fibrous and should be terminated. This limits the dissection just cephalad to the juxtaposed zygomatic nerve branches, which are commonly situated in the plane between the SMAS and the deep fascia in this location.
- Dissection anteriorly along the superior malar eminence, superficial to the zygomaticus major, is essential for malar pad repositioning. Facial nerve branches are protected in the region directly overlying the zygoma.
- Inferiorly, dissecting the lateral boarder of the platysma free from its ligamentous attachments to the anterior boarder of the SCM is important in providing adequate flap mobility. Once the SMAS/platysma is free from the SCM, an areolar plane is encountered. This areolar plane can be dissected bluntly, minimizing risk to the underlying cervical and marginal branches (►**Fig. 8.3**).

8.2 Technical Points: Extended SMAS Dissection

- The incision design for an extended SMAS dissection laterally parallels the zygomatic arch, which places the SMAS incision caudal to the path of the frontal branch.
- Anteriorly, in the region where the zygomatic arch joins the lateral zygoma, the SMAS incision courses superiorly along the superior boarder of the malar fat pad. The junction between the superior malar fat and the lateral orbicularis oculi (which is flat and has little overlying fat) is obvious in most patients, and marks the superior or "high" segment of the extended SMAS dissection. The lateral/inferior SMAS incision follows the lateral boarder of the platysma inferiorly in the neck, extending several centimeters caudal to the earlobe (►**Fig. 8.1**).
- Before dissecting the SMAS, hydrodissection with a small amount of local anesthetic is helpful. Once the SMAS is incised, the underlying parotid capsule with be noted. Defining the plane between the SMAS and the parotid capsule is important in setting the proper depth of dissection (►**Fig. 8.2**).
- The lateral boarder of the platysma is incised. The lateral platysma is usually thick and easy to dissect. Once the platysma is dissected past the restraint of the ligaments along the anterior boarder of the SCM, an areolar plane anterior to the SCM is encountered, and the inferior SMAS/platysma can be mobilized with blunt dissection.
- The SMAS in the malar area overlying the malar eminence and zygomaticus major is thick and fibrous as the zygomatic ligaments percolate through the malar fat pad. The plane between the zygomaticus major and the malar pad is typically easy to define and safe to dissect, as there are no facial nerve branches in this region (►**Fig. 8.2b**).
- Lateral to the zygoma, the SMAS is thin and easy to tear during dissection. In this region, the upper masseteric ligaments are encountered as well as the transverse facial perforator. To ensure adequate mobility of the lower cheek and jowl, release of the upper masseteric ligaments is

required. Proceed carefully in this region, recognizing the appearance of the ligaments and the thickness of the SMAS. If the plane of dissection is obscure, STOP, as the zygomatic branches are in close proximity in this region (▶ **Fig. 8.2b**).

- The transverse facial artery is an important landmark. Cephalad to this perforator there are no facial nerve branches, while distal to the artery the zygomatic nerve branches are in close proximity. Typically, the upper masseteric ligaments are just caudal to this artery, and only a few millimeters of distal dissection is required to reach the mobile region of the SMAS, past the restraint of the upper masseteric ligaments.
- In terms of the limits of SMAS dissection, the junction between the fixed and mobile region of the SMAS should be reached. The junction between fixed and mobile SMAS lies directly anterior to the parotid gland, anterior to the accessory lobe of the parotid, anterior/inferior to the lateral malar eminence, and anterior to the SCM (▶ **Fig. 8.3**).
- Flap mobility can be tested by traction on the SMAS flap and by judging unrestricted anterior cheek movement.
  - REMEMBER: when the dissection has proceeded into the mobile region of the SMAS, the dissection becomes easy and is no longer fibrous.
  - When the DISSECTION BECOMES EASY, STOP. This ensures adequate flap mobility as well as protection against inadvertent motor branch injury.

8.3 Dissection

- The incision of the SMAS is marked just cephalad to the zygomatic arch, which is a region directly overlying the parotid and caudal to the path of the frontal branch. The junction of the zygomatic arch with the body of the zygoma is marked, and at this point the SMAS incision continues along the superior border of the malar pad.
- To ensure that the SMAS dissection is caudal to the path of the frontal branch, an important step in preventing frontal branch injury is to mark a line from the tragus to the brow and to limit the SMAS incision caudal to this landmark. The lateral border of the platysma is marked inferiorly in the neck. The SMAS is infiltrated with local anesthesia to help with the hydrodissection.
- The SMAS elevation begins sharply overlying the parotid gland, identifying the interface between the parotid capsule and the SMAS. Dissection into parotid parenchyma should be avoided.
- The dissection is continued along the lateral border of the platysma inferiorly into the neck, several cm below the earlobe,
- The dissection is then carried along the undersurface of the platysma, freeing the platsyma from attachments to the SCM. The SMAS is elevated just anterior to the tail of the parotid and anterior to the retaining ligaments along the anterior border of the sternocleidomastoid muscle, where an areolar plane is identified. At this point, the mobilization of the lower SMAS/platyysma is completed with blunt dissection.
- Anterior to the tail of the parotid, sub-SMAS fat is identified, which is an important landmark, as this is the region where the marginal mandibular branch exits the parotid. Dissection in this region should proceed bluntly, with care to dissect superficial to the deep fascia.
  - Dissection superiorly along the main body of the parotid is carried toward its anterior boarder to ensure ligamentous release.

- Once the anterior border of the parotid is reached, sub-SMAS fat typically becomes visible, the mobile region of the SMAS is encountered, and the dissection terminated.
  - The surgeon will note that anterior to the parotid sub-SMAS dissection becomes less fibrous as the SMAS has been released from the retaining ligaments. As emphasized, when the dissection becomes easy, STOP. Further dissection does not increase flap mobility and serves only to increase the morbidity of the surgery.
  - From a safety perspective, the facial nerve branches are more exposed in the mobile region of the cheek, which is another reason to limit dissection once the SMAS flap has been mobilized.
- The malar extension of the SMAS dissection, to reposition the malar fat pad, carries the SMAS dissection over the lateral zygoma. The malar pad is then dissected free from its attachments to the zygoma, in the plane between the malar pad and the zygomaticus major.
- When elevating the malar pad, the fibers of the zygomaticus major (and more anteriorly the orbicularis oculi and zygomaticus minor) are visualized. These muscles are innervated along their deep surfaces, such that as the extended SMAS dissection is carried superficially to these muscles, motor branch injury will be prevented. The SMAS is elevated until the flap is freed from the underlying lateral zygomatic ligaments. The more medial malar dissection is then connected with the cheek SMAS flap dissection lateral to the zygomatic eminience, where the upper masseteric ligaments will be encountered.
- This portion of the SMAS dissection is performed at the end of SMAS flap elevation (following dissection of the SMAS over both the parotid and malar regions) to aid in correctly identifying the proper plane of dissection. During SMAS elevation, leaving sub-SMAS fat intact overlying the deep fascia provides increased protection against motor branch injury.

8.4 Lateral SMASectomy/Platysma Window Key Points

- In performing lateral SMASectomy, the junction between the fixed and mobile SMAS is identified. This junction is marked from just anterior to the tail of the parotid cephalically toward the lateral malar eminence (►Fig. 8.4).
- An elliptical excision of SMAS/superficial fat is designed based on removing redundant facial fat to correction facial laxity (►Fig. 8.5).
- The major advantage of the lateral SMASectomy technique is that it provides for facial fat repositioning without formal sub-SMAS dissection. To be effective, the caudal extent of the SMAS excision must be along the mobile region of the SMAS.
- In performing lateral SMASectomy, the superficial fascia is incised. Care is taken to perform the resection of SMAS just deep to the superficial fascia. The key to safety in performing lateral SMASectomy is to not violate the underlying deep facial fascia and parotid capsule, avoiding both nerve injury and parotid fistula.
- The platysma window technique frequently accompanies the lateral SMASectomy procedure, providing contouring of the jawline and neck. Unlike the technique of lateral SMASectomy, which has no formal

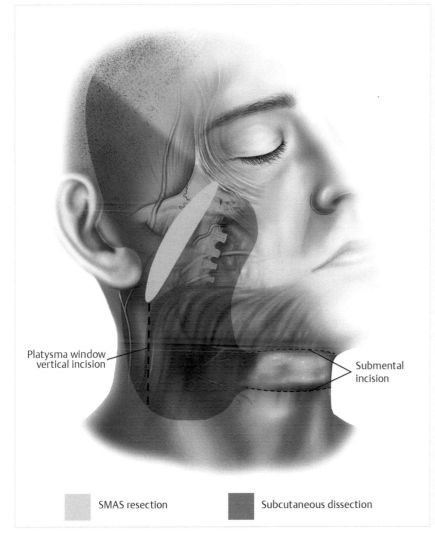

Platysma window
vertical incision

Submental
incision

SMAS resection

Subcutaneous dissection

Fig. 8.4 The incision design for lateral SMASectomy parallels the anterior boarder of the parotid, extending cephalad toward the malar eminence. This incision design represents the junction between the fixed and mobile regions of the SMAS and is similar in terms of the limits of dissection noted in an Extended SMAS dissection. If the platysma window is preformed in conjunction with lateral SMASectomy, the lateral boarder of the platysma is incised and dissected free from the retaining ligaments along the anterior boarder of the SCM.

sub-SMAS undermining, the platysma window technique requires an incision of the lateral boarder of the platysma extending from the earlobe caudally several cm inferiorly in the neck.

- Following platysma incision, the platysma is dissected from the retaining ligaments along the anterior boarder of the SCM. Typically, only a few cm of anterior dissection is required to obtain mobility, and once the areolar plane is reached anterior to the SCM, the dissection may be performed bluntly. The platysma window technique is analogous to the lateral/inferior dissection of the extended SMAS technique discussed previously (▶ Fig. 8.3).

8.5 Lateral SMASectomy/Platysma Window: Safety Considerations

- In performing lateral SMASectomy, the junction between the fixed and mobile SMAS is marked (▶ Fig. 8.4).
- The mobile SMAS, which is anterior to the parotid, represents a region where the facial nerve is less protected.

- When preforming SMAS excision, define the plane between the SMAS and deep fascia. Blunt dissection just deep to the SMAS following SMAS incision is useful in identifying the proper plane of excision. Perform the SMAS excision superficial to the deep fascia.
- Leaving sub-SMAS fat intact on the deep fascia protects underlying motor branches during SMAS excision.
- In performing lateral SMAS excision, do not violate the parotid capsule or dissect within the parotid parenchymal to avoid parotid fistula (►Fig. 8.5).
- In the lateral SMASectomy technique, the redundant fat can either be excised, as typical in heavy patients or left in place to add lateral cheek volume (termed SMAS stacking) which is appropriate in thin patients. Both procedures reposition facial fat as the SMASectomy incision lines are sutured (**Videos 8.1–8.3**).
- In performing a platysma window, when dissecting the lateral boarder of the platysma from its attachments to the SCM, dissect directly along the undersurface of the platysma to avoid injuring the great auricular nerve, which can be located close to the lateral platysma. When the platysma is freed from the SCM, an areolar plane will be encountered, and further dissection anteriorly should be performed bluntly to avoid cervical branch injury.

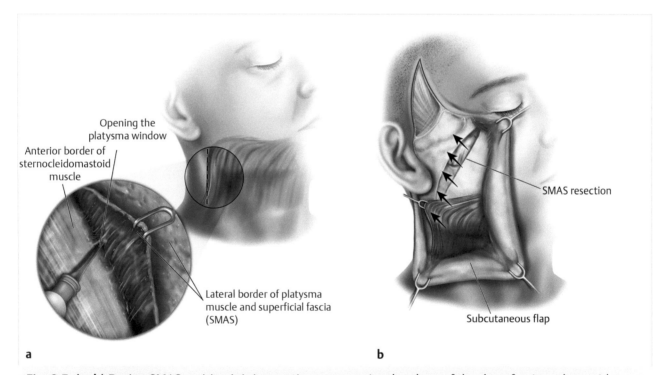

a

b

Fig. 8.5 (a, b) During SMAS excision it is imperative to recognize the plane of the deep fascia and parotid capsule and ensure the resection is superficial to these structures. Following SMAS excision the superficial fascia is carefully repaired, repositioning facial fat into the lateral cheek as appropriate in heavy patients. In thin patients, the redundant SMAS is left in place to add volume to the lateral cheek following incision closure. If the platysma window has been performed in conjunction with lateral SMASectomy, the platysma is fixated superior/laterally to the mastoid fascia.

8.6 Dissection Lateral Smasectomy: Technical Considerations

- The lateral SMASectomy technique involves an elliptical SMAS excision, which is designed at the junction between the mobile and the fixed SMAS.
- Following SMAS excision, the anterior facial fat is repositioned toward the suture line, which aids in tightening the lower cheek and elevating the malar pad.
- To be effective, the junction of the fixed and mobile SMAS must be recognized, and the incision design for a lateral SMASectomy is similar to the anterior limits for an extended SMAS dissection (the anterior border of the parotid, the upper masseteric ligaments, and lateral zygoma).
- For this reason, the elliptical incision is designed from the base of the earlobe to the superior aspect of the malar eminence.
- Following the design of the elliptical excision, the superficial fascia is infiltrated with local anesthesia. The surgeon then resects the superficial fascia within the ellipse, utilizing blunt dissection to identify the plane between superficial and deep fascia.
- Care to leave the underlying sub-SMAS fat intact overlying the deep fascia provides an element of protection against injury to deeply situated facial nerve branches. It is also important when performing a lateral SMASectomy to not dissect into the parotid parenchyma, specifically in the region of the tail of the parotid, to avoid an inadvertent parotid fistula. Similarly, superficial excision in the region lateral to the zygoma is stressed as the zygomatic branches are superficially positioned in this location.
- The redundant SMAS between the excision lines may be excised or left in place depending on the volumetric needs of the patient. In heavy patients, the SMAS is typically excised, while in thin patients, the SMAS is stacked to add volume in the lateral cheek (**Video 8.4**).
- The platysma window frequently accompanies the lateral SMASectomy technique, as it provides contouring of the jawline and neck. The incision and dissection in the platysma window technique is analogous to the lateral/inferior dissection of the platysma in the extendend SMAS dissection. Once the platysma is freed from the retaining ligaments along the anterior boarder of the SCM, the platysma is rotated superior/laterally and sutured to the mastoid fascia with care to span the path of the great auricular nerve (**Video 8.5**).

Suggested Readings

Aston S, Walden J. Facelift with Smas technique and FAE. In: Aston S, Steinbrech D, Walden J, eds. Aesthetic Plastic Surgery. London, Saunders Elsevier; 2009

Baker DC. Lateral SMASectomy. Plast Reconstr Surg. 1997; 100(2):509–513

Baker DC. Minimal incision rhtyidectomy with lateral SMASectomy. Aesthet Surg J. 2001; 21:68

Baker TJ, Gordon HL, Stuzin JM. Surgical Rejuvenation of the Face. 2nd ed. St Louis, Mosby Year-Book; 1996

Barton FE, Jr. The SMAS and the nasolabial fold. Plast Reconstr Surg. 1992; 89(6):1054–1057, discussion 1058–1059

Connell B. Marten, T the trifurcated SMAS flap for improved results in the midface, cheek, and neck. Aesthetic Plast Surg. 1995; 19:415

Hamra ST. The deep-plane rhytidectomy. Plast Reconstr Surg. 1990; 86(1):53–61, discussion 62–63

Lemmon ML. Superficial fascia rhytidectomy. A restoration of the SMAS with control of the cervicomental angle. Clin Plast Surg. 1983; 10(3):449–478

Marten TJ. High SMAS facelift: combined single flap lifting of the jawline, cheek, and midface. Clin Plast Surg. 2008; 35(4):569–603, vi–vii

Mendelson BC. Surgery of the superficial musculoaponeurotic system: principles of release, vectors, and fixation. Plast Reconstr Surg. 2001; 107(6):1545–1552, discussion 1553–1555, 1556–1557, 1558–1561

Owsley JQ, Jr. Platysma-fascial rhytidectomy: a preliminary report. Plast Reconstr Surg. 1977; 60(6):843–850

Owsley JQ. Lifting the malar fat pad for correction of prominent nasolabial folds. Plast Reconstr Surg. 1993; 91(3):463–474, discussion 475–476

Rohrich RJ, Narasimhan K. Long-Term Results in Face Lifting: Observational Results and Evolution of Technique. Plast Reconstr Surg. 2016; 138(1):97–108

Stuzin JM, Baker TJ, Gordon HL, Baker TM. Extended SMAS dissection as an approach to midface rejuvenation. Clin Plast Surg. 1995; 22(2):295–311

Stuzin JM. Restoring facial shape in face lifting: the role of skeletal support in facial analysis and midface soft-tissue repositioning. Plast Reconstr Surg. 2007; 119(1):362–376, discussion 377–378

Stuzin JM. MOC-PSSM CME article: Face lifting. Plast Reconstr Surg. 2008; 121(1, Suppl):1–19

Tonnard P, Verpaele A, Monstrey S, et al. Minimal access cranial suspension lift: a modified S-lift. Plast Reconstr Surg. 2002; 109(6):2074–2086

Part II

Fillers and Neuromodulators

*Rod J .Rohrich, Dinah Wan,
and Raja Mohan*

9 Introduction

Rod J. Rohrich and Dinah Wan

Abstract
Inadvertent injury to facial vessels during the injection of facial fillers or neuro-modulators may lead to undesirable consequences. Proper anatomical knowledge of the rich vascular networks of the face and the execution of safe injection techniques are critical in providing optimal outcomes.

Keywords: facial danger zones, injection technique, intravascular injection

While the neural anatomy, specifically the branches of the facial nerve, are of primary interest when describing facial zones at risk for injury during facelift procedures,[1,2] vascular anatomy becomes principally important in the discussion of nonsurgical facial injection techniques. The utmost concern with injectables is inadvertent violation of the exceptionally rich vascular network of the face. Intravascular injection of foreign material incurs consequences ranging from benign bruising to more threatening complications such as tissue necrosis, blindness, stroke, and even death.[3]

In Part II, we describe the facial danger zones with respect to injection of fillers and neuromodulators, focusing on specific facial vessels at risk for inadvertent cannulation and anatomical landmarks used to identify these vessels. We also discuss safe injection techniques specific to each of the six facial danger zones, including the following (▶ Fig. 9.1):

1. Glabellar region
2. Temporal region
3. Perioral region
4. Nasolabial region
5. Nasal region
6. Infraorbital region

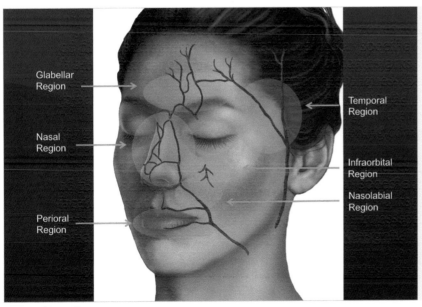

Fig. 9.1 The six vascular danger zones of the face and associated at-risk vessels.

9.1 General Safety Principles

Anatomic region aside, the following general safety principles should remain at the core of every facial injection technique[4,5,6]:

- Use reversible fillers (i.e., hyaluronic acid).
- Use epinephrine or ice for vasoconstriction.
- Use small syringes (0.5 to 1 mL) and inject in small increments.
- Use small needles (27 G or smaller).
- Use cannulas when appropriate.
- Use anterograde–retrograde injection.
- Use constant, steady, slow motion.
- Use low-pressure injection; injections requiring high pressure indicate danger and/or inappropriate location.
- Use caution when injecting in areas of previous trauma, as tissue planes may be scarred and obscured.
- Be aware of pertinent anatomy of the vascular danger zones.
- Have a filler rescue kit available at all times (hyaluronidase, aspirin, nitroglycerin ointment).

References

[1] Seckel BR. Facial Danger Zones: Avoiding nerve injury in facial plastic surgery. 2nd ed. New York, NY: Thieme Medical Publishers, Inc.; 2010

[2] Roostaeian J, Rohrich RJ, Stuzin JM. Anatomical considerations to prevent facial nerve injury. Plast Reconstr Surg. 2015; 135(5):1318–1327

[3] Scheuer JF, III, Sieber DA, Pezeshk RA, Gassman AA, Campbell CF, Rohrich RJ. Facial Danger Zones: Techniques to Maximize Safety during Soft-Tissue Filler Injections. Plast Reconstr Surg. 2017; 139(5):1103–1108

[4] Scheuer JF, III, Sieber DA, Pezeshk RA, Campbell CF, Gassman AA, Rohrich RJ. Anatomy of the Facial Danger Zones: Maximizing Safety during Soft-Tissue Filler Injections. Plast Reconstr Surg. 2017; 139(1):50e–58e

[5] Kurkjian TJ, Ahmad J, Rohrich RJ. Soft-tissue fillers in rhinoplasty. Plast Reconstr Surg. 2014; 133(2):121e–126e

[6] Rohrich RJ. Personal Communication. Nov 2017

10 Facial Danger Zone 1– Glabellar Region

Rod J. Rohrich and Dinah Wan

Abstract

The glabellar region is the most common filler injection site leading to blindness due to the rich anastomotic network between the supratrochlear, supraorbital, and dorsal nasal arteries. Inadvertent injection into any of these arteries can create retrograde embolus into the ophthalmic artery. The supratrochlear artery courses very superficially, often within the glabellar frown crease. Injections in the glabellar rhytides should be performed very superficially within the dermis using serial puncture technique and low pressure. Digital pressure should be applied at the supraorbital rim to occlude the supratrochlear and supraorbital vessels while injecting in the glabella.

Keywords: filler injection, glabellar frown lines, supraorbital artery, supratrochlear artery, blindness

---

Key Points for Maximizing Filler Safety in the Glabellar Region

- Use fillers primarily for **superficial line-filling** in the glabellar area.
- Use **serial puncture** technique to deposit small aliquots **intradermally** along rhytids.
- Use digital pressure to **occlude the supraorbital and supratrochlear vessels** at the supraorbital rim.
- Do not attempt to overcorrect deep rhytids in the glabellar region.

10.1 Safety Considerations in the Glabellar Region

- The glabella has been reported as the most common filler injection site leading to blindness, and the second most common for skin necrosis.[1,2,3,4,5]
- Rich anastomoses exist between the supratrochlear, supraorbital, and dorsal nasal arteries, all of which are branches of the ophthalmic artery (▶ **Fig. 10.1a**).
- Inadvertent intravascular injection into the nasoglabellar arcade can create retrograde propagation of foreign material into the ophthalmic artery (▶ **Fig. 10.1b**).
- Subsequent distal embolism from the ophthalmic artery can cause vision loss and/or tissue necrosis.[6,7]

10.2 Pertinent Anatomy of the Brow and Glabellar Region

A cadaveric dissection showing pertinent arteries and muscles in the glabellar and brow region is shown in ▶ **Fig. 10.2**.

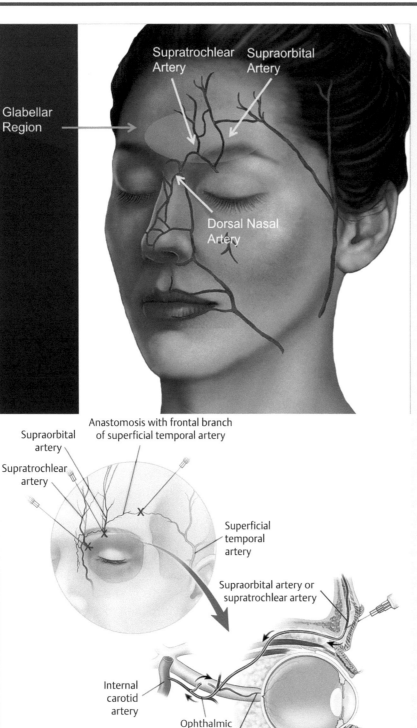

Fig. 10.1 (a) Rich anastomoses between the supratrochlear, supraorbital, and dorsal nasal arteries in the glabellar region create potential routes for retrograde embolization to the ophthalmic artery. (b) Inadvertent intravascular injection into the supraorbital or supratrochlear artery can create retrograde propagation of foreign material into the ophthalmic artery. Subsequent distal embolism from the ophthalmic artery into the central retinal artery can cause vision loss.

10.2.1 Arteries (▶Fig. 10.3)

Supratrochlear Artery

- A branch of the ophthalmic artery.
- Exits the superomedial orbit in-line with the median canthus +/- 3 mm, or 17 to 22 mm lateral to midline.[8,9,10,11]
- Traverses vertically through the corrugator, then through the frontalis and orbicularis to enter the subcutaneous plane 15 to 25 mm above the orbital rim.[9]
- Continues superiorly in paramedian forehead in the subcutaneous plane, 15 to 20 mm from midline.[10]

Supraorbital Artery

- A branch of the ophthalmic artery.
- Exits the superior orbit in-line with the medial limbus, or 32 mm lateral to midline.[9,11]
- Pierces the frontalis 20 to 40 mm above the orbital rim and emerges in the subcutaneous plane 40 to 60 mm above the orbital rim.[12]

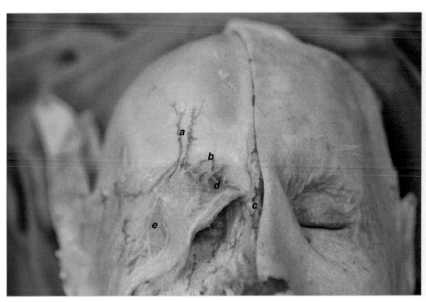

Fig. 10.2 The supraorbital artery **(a)** is shown exiting above the brow, ramifying a periosteal branch before traversing the subgaleal plane. The supratrochlear artery **(b)** lies medial, piercing the corrugator muscle **(d)**, and anastomosing with the dorsal nasal artery **(c)** and the supraorbital artery **(a)**. The frontalis muscle **(e)** is reflected up with galea and seen on its undersurface.

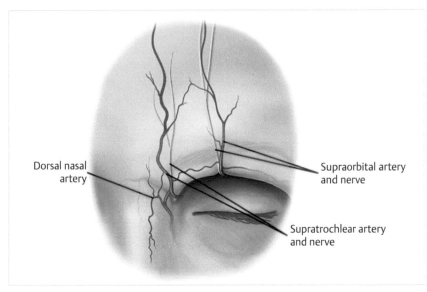

Dorsal nasal artery

Supraorbital artery and nerve

Supratrochlear artery and nerve

Fig. 10.3 Diagram showing the major neurovascular structures in the glabellar region. The supratrochlear artery and nerve exit the superomedial orbit in-line with the medial canthus. The supraorbital artery and nerve exit the superior obit in-line with the medial limbus. The dorsal nasal artery emerges from the medial orbit and courses over the nasal radix caudally toward the nasal tip.

Dorsal Nasal Artery

- A terminal branch of the ophthalmic artery.
- Emerges from the medial orbit.
- Courses medially over the nasal radix above the muscular layer, then continues caudally toward the nasal tip.[13]

10.2.2 Muscles (▶ Fig. 10.4a)

Corrugator Supercilii

- Originates on the nasal process of the frontal bone.
- Inserts superolaterally into the dermis of the brow.
- Responsible for vertical and oblique glabellar frown lines.

Procerus

- Originates on the lower part of the nasal bone.
- Inserts into the forehead dermis between the eyebrows.
- Responsible for transverse dorsal nasal rhytids, or "bunny lines."

Frontalis

- Originates from the frontal galea aponeurotica.
- Interdigitates with the orbicularis oculi, procerus, and corrugator muscle fibers at the brow.
- Responsible for transverse forehead rhytids.

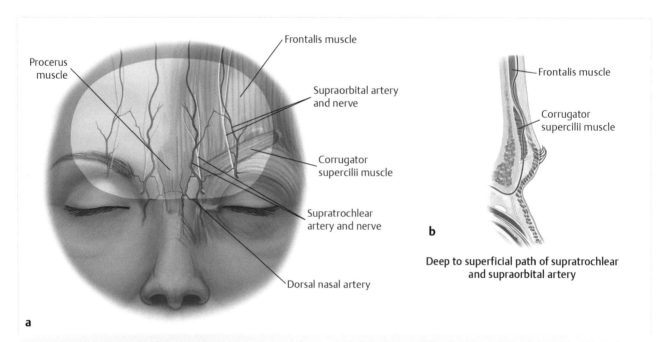

Fig. 10.4 (a) Diagram showing the mimetic muscles in the glabellar and forehead region. The corrugator supercilii muscle is responsible for vertical and oblique glabellar frown lines. The procerus muscle is responsible for transverse dorsal nasal rhytids. The frontalis muscle is responsible for transverse forehead rhytids. **(b)** Cross section demonstrating the deep-to-superficial path of the supratrochlear and supraorbital artery as it exits the supraorbital rim.

10.3 Vascular Danger Zones and Clinical Correlations

- **Arteries in the glabellar region** *quickly become superficial* after arising from the orbit and often closely abut skin rhytids, thus making them vulnerable to injury even with relatively superficial injections (►Fig. 10.4b).
- This is especially true for the supratrochlear artery, which lies *within* the glabellar frown line in 50% of cases (►Fig. 10.5).[14]
- Anatomic variations of the supraorbital artery also make it vulnerable to injury, as it transitions from the submuscular to the subcutaneous plane at variable distances above the orbital rim and may give off superficial branches as low as 15 mm above the rim.[9,12]
- The dorsal nasal artery courses over the nasal radix in the subdermal plane just below the transverse nasal rhytids, thus creating another zone of potential vascular compromise when injecting the bunny lines with fillers. In this region, injections should be performed close to midline in the preperichondrial or preperiosteal plane, staying *deep* to vulnerable vessels.[1,7,13]
- **Occluding the supraorbital and supratrochlear vessels** with digital pressure at the orbital rim prevents retrograde flow of foreign material into the ophthalmic artery in the event of inadvertent intravascular injection (►Fig. 10.6) (**Video 10.1**).

10.4 Technical Points for Filler Injection in the Glabellar Region

- Inject filler **very superficially** when treating glabellar rhytids to avoid disrupting the rich subcutaneous vascular network in the region.

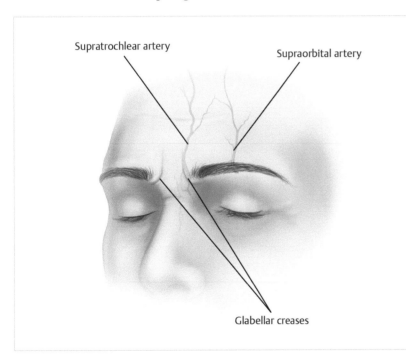

Fig. 10.5 The supratrochlear artery quickly becomes superficial after exiting the orbit and often closely abuts the glabellar frown lines directly under the dermis.

Supratrochlear artery

Supraorbital artery

Glabellar creases

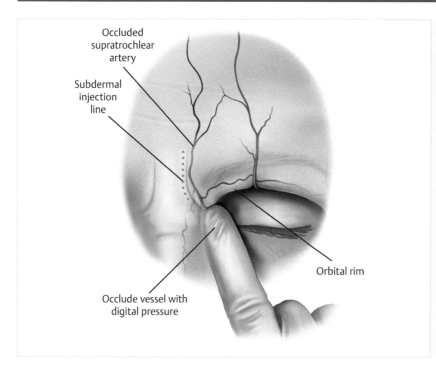

Fig. 10.6 The supratrochlear artery is occluded with digital pressure at the superomedial orbital rim to prevent retrograde flow of foreign material into the ophthalmic artery in the event of inadvertent intravascular injection.

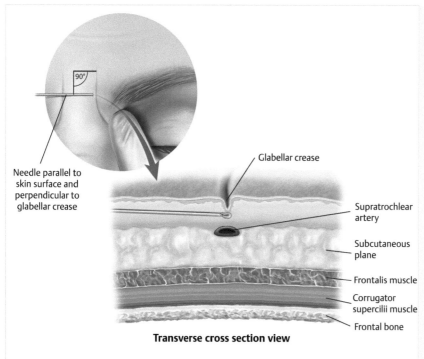

Fig. 10.7 Glabellar frown lines should be injected using serial puncture technique with small aliquots deposited intradermally at a 90° angle to the glabellar crease.

- Use a **low-G'** filler to prevent the Tyndall effect.
- Use **serial puncture** technique with small aliquots deposited **intradermally** along rhytids at a 90° angle to the glabellar crease (▶**Fig. 10.7**) (**Video 10.2**).
- Perform **low-pressure** injections.
- **Apply digital pressure at the supraorbital rim** to occlude the supraorbital and supratrochlear vessels while injecting in the glabella.

References

[1] Scheuer JF, III, Sieber DA, Pezeshk RA, Campbell CF, Gassman AA, Rohrich RJ. Anatomy of the Facial Danger Zones: Maximizing Safety during Soft-Tissue Filler Injections. Plast Reconstr Surg. 2017; 139(1):50e–58e

[2] Li X, Du L, Lu JJ. A Novel Hypothesis of Visual Loss Secondary to Cosmetic Facial Filler Injection. Ann Plast Surg. 2015; 75(3):258–260

[3] Ozturk CN, Li Y, Tung R, Parker L, Piliang MP, Zins JE. Complications following injection of soft-tissue fillers. Aesthet Surg J. 2013; 33(6):862–877

[4] Park KH, Kim YK, Woo SJ, et al; Korean Retina Society. Iatrogenic occlusion of the ophthalmic artery after cosmetic facial filler injections: a national survey by the Korean Retina Society. JAMA Ophthalmol. 2014; 132(6):714–723

[5] Park SW, Woo SJ, Park KH, Huh JW, Jung C, Kwon OK. Iatrogenic retinal artery occlusion caused by cosmetic facial filler injections. Am J Ophthalmol. 2012; 154(4):653–662.e1

[6] Carruthers JD, Fagien S, Rohrich RJ, Weinkle S, Carruthers A. Blindness caused by cosmetic filler injection: a review of cause and therapy. Plast Reconstr Surg. 2014; 134(6):1197–1201

[7] Scheuer JF, III, Sieber DA, Pezeshk RA, Gassman AA, Campbell CF, Rohrich RJ. Facial Danger Zones: Techniques to Maximize Safety during Soft-Tissue Filler Injections. Plast Reconstr Surg. 2017; 139(5):1103–1108

[8] Ugur MB, Savranlar A, Uzun L, Küçüker H, Cinar F. A reliable surface landmark for localizing supratrochlear artery: medial canthus. Otolaryngol Head Neck Surg. 2008; 138(2):162–165

[9] Kleintjes WG. Forehead anatomy: arterial variations and venous link of the midline forehead flap. J Plast Reconstr Aesthet Surg. 2007; 60(6):593–606

[10] Shumrick KA, Smith TL. The anatomic basis for the design of forehead flaps in nasal reconstruction. Arch Otolaryngol Head Neck Surg. 1992; 118(4):373–379

[11] Webster RC, Gaunt JM, Hamdan US, Fuleihan NS, Giandello PR, Smith RC. Supraorbital and supratrochlear notches and foramina: anatomical variations and surgical relevance. Laryngoscope. 1986; 96(3):311–315

[12] Erdogmus S, Govsa F. Anatomy of the supraorbital region and the evaluation of it for the reconstruction of facial defects. J Craniofac Surg. 2007; 18(1):104–112

[13] Toriumi DM, Mueller RA, Grosch T, Bhattacharyya TK, Larrabee WF, Jr. Vascular anatomy of the nose and the external rhinoplasty approach. Arch Otolaryngol Head Neck Surg. 1996; 122(1):24–34

[14] Vural E, Batay F, Key JM. Glabellar frown lines as a reliable landmark for the supratrochlear artery. Otolaryngol Head Neck Surg. 2000; 123(5):543–546

11 Facial Danger Zone 2 – Temporal Region

Rod J. Rohrich and Dinah Wan

Abstract
The superficial temporal artery and middle temporal vein lie within the temporal fossa in an intermediate plane. Inadvertent injection into the frontal branch of the superficial temporal artery can cause ocular compromise via retrograde embolization through the supraorbital system. Injection into the middle temporal vein may result in nonthrombotic pulmonary embolism via anterograde venous flow into the internal jugular vein. Filler injections in the temporal region should be performed either superficially in the subcutaneous tissue, or deeply in the preperiosteal plane to avoid inadvertent cannulation of at-risk vessels situated in the intermediate plane.

Keywords: filler injections, temporal fossa, frontal branch of superficial temporal artery, middle temporal vein, blindness, pulmonary embolus

---

Key Points for Maximizing Filler Safety in the Temporal Region

- **Avoid injecting in the intermediate plane** where vulnerable vessels lie in the temporal region.
- Inject either superficially in the **superficial subcutaneous** tissue or deeply in the **preperiosteal** plane.
- Inject with low pressure in an anterograde/retrograde motion.

11.1 Safety Considerations in the Temporal Region

- The superficial temporal artery and middle temporal vein lie within the temporal fossa in an intermediate plane (►**Fig. 11.1**).
- Intravascular injection of foreign material into the frontal branch of the superficial temporal artery can cause ocular compromise via retrograde embolization through the supraorbital system[1](►**Fig. 11.2**).
- Dye injected into the superficial temporal artery has been found within ipsilateral and even bilateral globes in cadaver studies.[2]
- Although extremely rare, intravascular injection into the middle temporal vein can cause nonthrombotic pulmonary embolism via anterograde venous flow into the internal jugular vein.[3,4]

11.2 Pertinent Anatomy of the Temporal Region

11.2.1 Superficial Temporal Artery – Frontal Branch (►Fig. 11.3) (Video 11.1)

- Path is similar to the temporal branch of the facial nerve.
- Originates 1 fingerbreadth anterior and 2 fingerbreadths superior to the tip of the tragus.[5]
- Runs in the intermediate plane within temporoparietal fascia 2 cm above zygomatic arch.[1,6]
- Transitions to the subcutaneous plane 1 fingerbreadth superior to the peak of the brow near the lateral border of the frontalis.[1]
- Anastomoses with the supraorbital artery above the lateral brow.

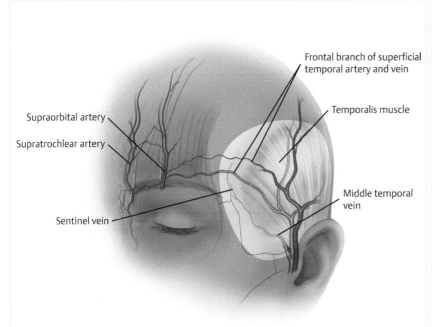

Fig. 11.1 The frontal branch of the superficial temporal artery and the middle temporal vein are potential sites of vascular injury during injections in the temporal region.

Frontal branch of superficial temporal artery and vein

Temporalis muscle

Supraorbital artery

Supratrochlear artery

Middle temporal vein

Sentinel vein

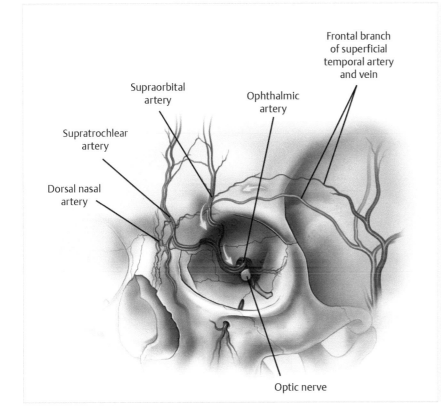

Fig. 11.2 The frontal branch of the superficial temporal artery lies in the temporal fossa and is at risk for inadvertent cannulation during injection in the temporal region. This branch arborizes with the supraorbital vessels in the lateral brow, creating potential routes for retrograde embolization into the ophthalmic system.

Frontal branch of superficial temporal artery and vein

Supraorbital artery

Ophthalmic artery

Supratrochlear artery

Dorsal nasal artery

Optic nerve

11.2.2 Middle Temporal Vein (▶Fig. 11.3)

- Runs 20 mm above and parallel to the zygomatic arch (**Fig. 9.4a**).[7]
- In the superficial temporal fat pad (▶**Fig. 11.4b**).
- Average size is 5 mm, can be as large as 9 mm.
- Connections with sentinel vein and cavernous sinus.
- Anterograde drainage into the internal jugular vein.[8]

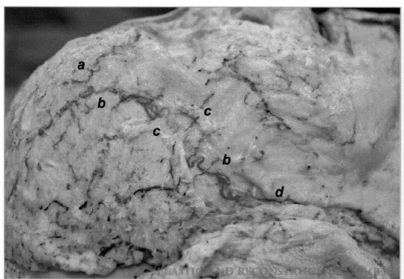

Fig. 11.3 The superficial temporal artery **(d)** is demonstrated ramifying its frontal branch **(b)**. The subcutaneous tissue **(c)** has been reflected anteriorly and posteriorly to delineate the course of the frontal branch artery within the superficial temporal fascia. The frontal branch artery **(b)** can be clearly seen anastomosing with the supraorbital artery **(a)** superficial to the frontalis muscle after transitioning to the subcutaneous plane.

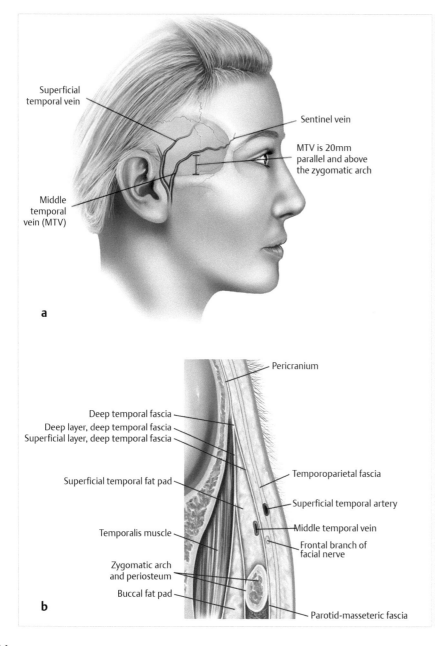

Fig. 11.4 The middle temporal vein runs 20 mm above and parallel to the zygomatic arch **(a)** and lies within the superficial temporal fat pad **(b)** at this level. It becomes more superficial as it travels toward the lateral brow where it has connections with the sentinel vein.

11.3 Vascular Danger Zones and Clinical Correlations

- At-risk vessels in the temporal region lie in an intermediate plane.
- Avoid injecting into the intermediate plane by placing filler either superficially just below the dermis, or deep in the preperiosteal plane.
- If injecting superficially, stay very superficial, just under the dermis, to avoid the frontal branch of the superficial temporal artery, which lies in a more intermediate plane.[1,5,8] Inject in an anterograde–retrograde fashion, maintaining the needle in an orientation almost parallel to the dermis (▶ Fig. 11.5) (Video 11.2).
- If injecting deep in the preperiosteal plane, stay within 1 fingerbreadth of the arch or greater than 25 mm above the arch to avoid inadvertent cannulation of the middle temporal vein (▶ Fig. 11.6).[1,7]

11.4 Technical Points for Filler Injection in the Temporal Region

- **Inject either deeply or superficially** in the temporal region. Avoid injecting in an intermediate depth.[1]
- If injecting superficially, inject in the **superficial subcutaneous tissue** just below the dermis (**Video 11.2**).
- Start at the pretrichial area and progress medially.
- Inject in a slow, **constant anterograde–retrograde motion**.
- Consider using a cannula to lessen the chance of vessel puncture.
- If injecting deeply, use a high-G' filler and inject in the **preperiosteal plane**, staying within 1 fingerbreadth of the arch or at least 2.5 cm above it.

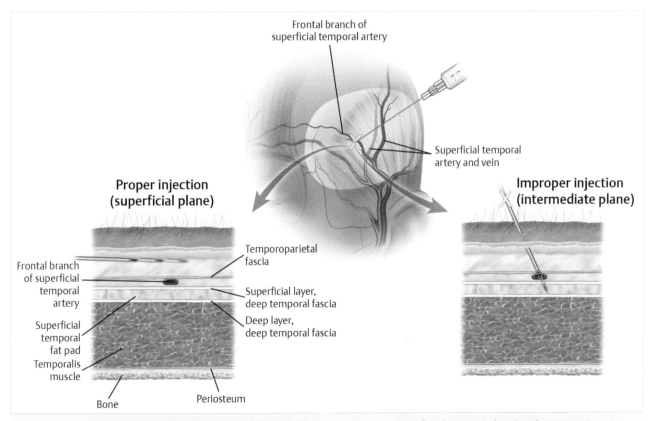

Fig. 11.5 If injecting superficially in the temporal region, stay very superficial, just under the dermis. Inject in an anterograde–retrograde fashion, maintaining the needle in an orientation almost parallel to the dermis.

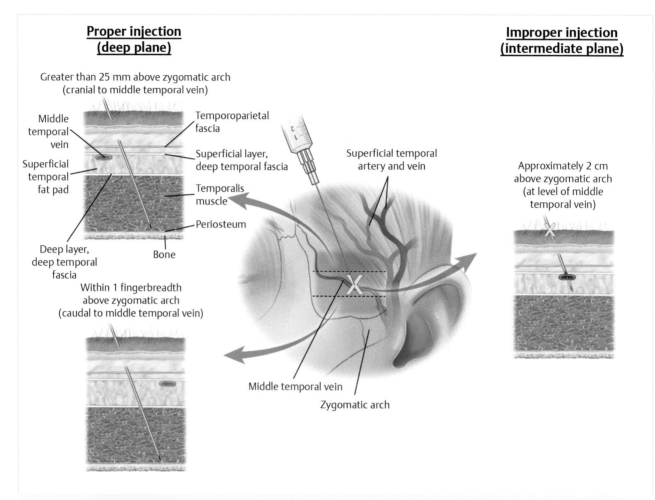

Fig. 11.6 If injecting deep in the preperiosteal plane, stay within 1 fingerbreadth of the arch or greater than 25 mm above the arch to avoid inadvertent cannulation of the middle temporal vein, which lies in a more intermediate plane approximately 20 mm above the zygomatic arch.

References

[1] Scheuer JF, III, Sieber DA, Pezeshk RA, Gassman AA, Campbell CF, Rohrich RJ. Facial Danger Zones: Techniques to Maximize Safety during Soft-Tissue Filler Injections. Plast Reconstr Surg. 2017; 139(5):1103–1108

[2] Tansatit T, Moon HJ, Apinuntrum P, Phetudom T. Verification of Embolic Channel Causing Blindness Following Filler Injection. Aesthetic Plast Surg. 2015; 39(1):154–161

[3] Jiang X, Liu DL, Chen B. Middle temporal vein: a fatal hazard in injection cosmetic surgery for temple augmentation. JAMA Facial Plast Surg. 2014; 16(3):227–229

[4] Jang JG, Hong KS, Choi EY. A case of nonthrombotic pulmonary embolism after facial injection of hyaluronic Acid in an illegal cosmetic procedure. Tuberc Respir Dis (Seoul). 2014; 77(2):90–93

[5] Lee JG, Yang HM, Hu KS, et al. Frontal branch of the superficial temporal artery: anatomical study and clinical implications regarding injectable treatments. Surg Radiol Anat. 2015; 37(1):61–68

[6] Trussler AP, Stephan P, Hatef D, Schaverien M, Meade R, Barton FE. The frontal branch of the facial nerve across the zygomatic arch: anatomical relevance of the high-SMAS technique. Plast Reconstr Surg. 2010; 125(4):1221–1229

[7] Jung W, Youn KH, Won SY, Park JT, Hu KS, Kim HJ. Clinical implications of the middle temporal vein with regard to temporal fossa augmentation. Dermatol Surg. 2014; 40(6):618–623

[8] Tansatit T, Apinuntrum P, Phetudom T. An Anatomical Study of the Middle Temporal Vein and the Drainage Vascular Networks to Assess the Potential Complications and the Preventive Maneuver During Temporal Augmentation Using Both Anterograde and Retrograde Injections. Aesthetic Plast Surg. 2015; 39(5):791–799

12 Facial Danger Zone 3 – Perioral Region

Rod J. Rohrich and Dinah Wan

Abstract
The superior and inferior labial arteries course within the upper and lower lips, respectively, in the deep plane between the orbicularis oris muscle and oral mucosa. Filler injections in the lips should remain superficial to the labial arteries to avoid excessive bruising. Injections should be performed no deeper than 3 mm from the vermilion or skin, within the subcutaneous or superficial intramuscular plane. The facial artery courses approximately 15 mm lateral to the oral commissure and is at risk for injury and subsequent distal embolus when injecting near the corner of the mouth. Injections in this region should be performed in the superficial subcutaneous tissue and within one thumbwidth of the commissure.

Keywords: filler injections, lips, oral commissure, corner of mouth, superior/ inferior labial artery, facial artery, tissue necrosis, bruising

---

Key Points for Maximizing Filler Safety in the Perioral Region

- Filler injections in the upper or lower lip should be placed **no deeper than 3 mm** from the skin or vermilion, within the **subcutaneous** or **superficial intramuscular** plane.
- Injections in the oral commissure should stay **within a thumbwidth** of the corner of mouth in the **superficial subcutaneous** plane.[1,2]
- Inject with low pressure in an anterograde/retrograde fashion.

12.1 Safety Considerations in the Perioral Region

- The superior and inferior labial arteries course within the upper and lower lips, respectively. Avoidance of these vessels when injecting filler for lip augmentation is critical to prevent tissue ischemia and/or excessive bruising (▶ Fig. 12.1).
- The facial artery courses just lateral to the oral commissure and is at risk for injury when injecting near the corner of the mouth.

12.2 Pertinent Anatomy of the Perioral Region

12.2.1 Upper Lip

Superior Labial Artery

- Originates from the facial artery 10 to 12 mm lateral to and 5 to 9 mm above commissure (▶ Fig. 12.2).[3,4,5,6]
- There is greater variability in the trajectory of the superior labial artery along the upper lip as compared to the path of the inferior labial artery in the lower lip.
- Initially runs superior to vermilion border along the lateral third of upper lip, then dips below border as it approaches the middle third or Cupid's bow.[6]

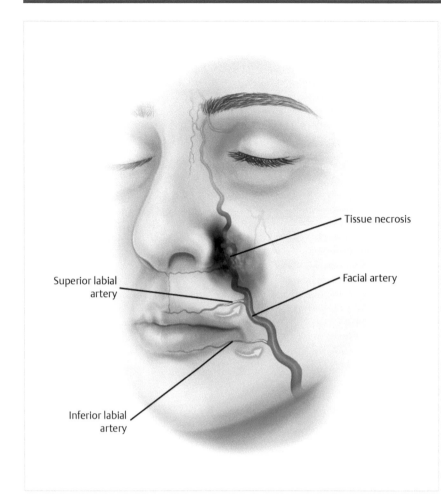

Tissue necrosis

Facial artery

Superior labial artery

Inferior labial artery

Fig. 12.1 The superior and inferior labial arteries' courses, respectively, within the upper and lower lips. These are at risk for injury during filler injections in the lips. The facial artery courses near the oral commissure as it gives off the labial artery branches and may be disrupted if injections are performed too laterally in the perioral region. Inadvertent injection of filler material into these vessels may lead to distal embolus and tissue necrosis in the angular artery region.

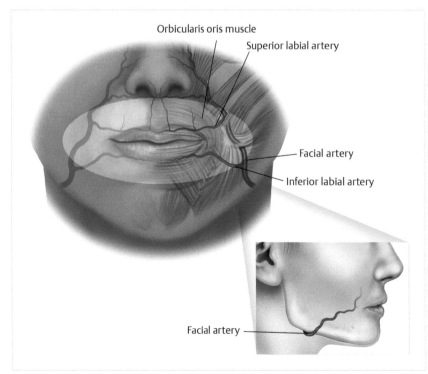

Orbicularis oris muscle

Superior labial artery

Facial artery

Inferior labial artery

Facial artery

Fig. 12.2 The superior labial artery originates from the facial artery lateral to and above the oral commissure, while the inferior labial artery more commonly branches from the facial artery inferolaterally to the oral commissure. The facial artery emerges from the angle of the mandible in the deep plane below the mimetic muscles and courses superficially toward the oral commissure.

- Courses 3 to 7.6 mm deep to the skin.[4,6]
- Most commonly found in the plane between the orbicularis oris and the oral mucosa, and less often within the orbicularis (▶ **Fig. 12.3**).[4,6,7]

12.2.2 Lower Lip

Inferior Labial Artery

- Variable origin due to inconsistent nomenclature, but typically branches from the facial artery inferolateral to the oral commissure (▶ **Fig. 12.2**).[1,4,5,8,9,10]
- Horizontal trajectory in the lower lip at the level of the vermilion/cutaneous junction.[8]
- Most commonly found in the plane between the orbicularis oris and the oral mucosa, and less often within the orbicularis (▶ **Fig. 12.3**).[7,9]

12.2.3 Oral Commissure

Facial Artery

- Emerges from the angle of the mandible in the deep plane below the mimetic muscles (▶ **Fig. 12.2**) (**Video 12.1**).
- Becomes more superficial and gives off the superior labial artery branch as it approaches the commissure.
- Located a thumbwidth, or 14 to 16 mm, lateral to the commissure.[6,9]

12.3 Vascular Danger Zones and Clinical Correlations

- The inferior and superior labial arteries lie in the plane between the orbicularis and the oral mucosa in 78.1% of cases, and within the orbicularis in 17.5%.[7]
- Labial artery depth is most variable in the central lip and can be found more frequently in superficial positions in the paramedian location.[7]
- Filler should be injected superficial to the labial arteries in the upper and lower lips. In general, this should be in the subcutaneous or superficial muscular plane, or no more than 3 mm deep to the skin (▶ **Fig. 12.4**).[1,2]

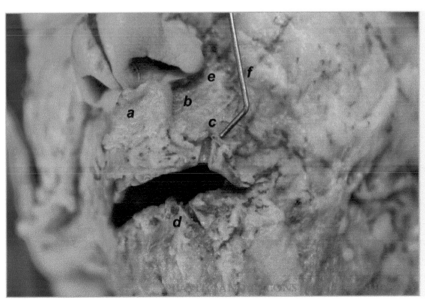

Fig. 12.3 Cadaveric dissection of the perioral region. The subcutaneous tissue (a) has been reflected, revealing the orbicularis oris muscle (b). The superior labial artery (c) can be seen running deep to the orbicularis on the labial mucosa, superior to the inferior lip border. The inferior labial artery (d) is demonstrated running in a similar fashion in the lower lip. The facial artery (f) is seen ramifying the inferior alar artery (e) in the upper third of the nasolabial fold.

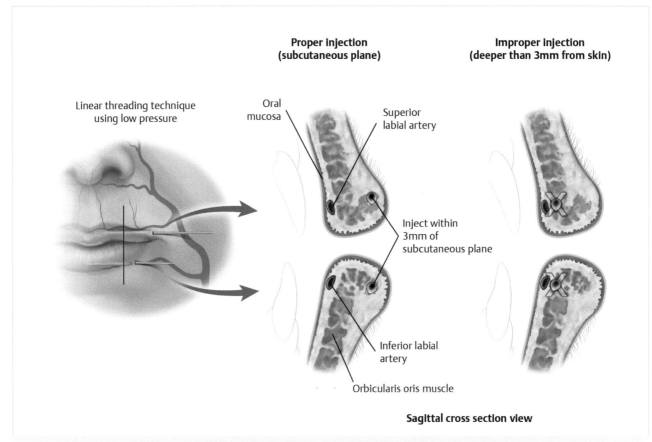

Fig. 12.4 Injections in the upper and lower lips. Filler should be injected superficially to the labial arteries in the upper and lower lips. In general, this should be in the subcutaneous or superficial orbicularis oris muscular plane, or no more than 3 mm deep to the skin.

- Stay more superficial when injecting filler in the midline lip, and avoid injecting the midpoint from commissure to Cupid's bow due to potentially more superficial vasculature in the paramedian lip.[7]
- Filler injection in the oral commissure should stay within the superficial plane within one thumbwidth from the corner of the mouth. Injecting filler too deeply or laterally from the corner of mouth (greater than one thumbwidth) risks violating the facial artery (▶ **Fig. 12.5**).[6,9]

12.4 Technical Points for Filler Injection in the Perioral Region

12.4.1 Upper and Lower Lip

- Use an intermediate or low-G' filler.[1,2]
- Use **linear threading** technique to inject along the vermilion/cutaneous border or within the dry vermilion[2,5,10] (**Video 12.2**).
- Use a gentle, low-pressure anterograde and retrograde maneuver.
- Inject *no deeper than 3 mm* in the subcutaneous or superficial intramuscular plane (▶ **Fig. 12.4**).[1,2,6]
- Consider staying more superficial in the central lip.[7]

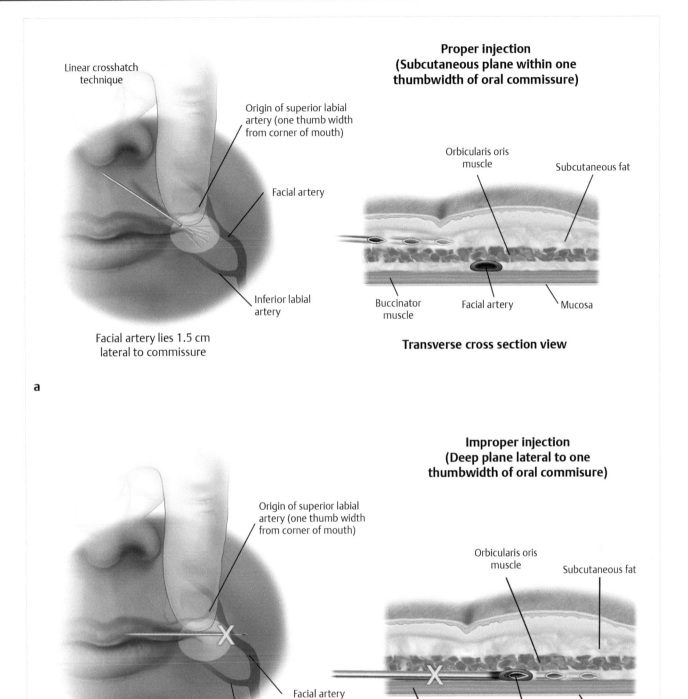

Linear crosshatch technique

Origin of superior labial artery (one thumb width from corner of mouth)

Facial artery

Inferior labial artery

Facial artery lies 1.5 cm lateral to commissure

Proper injection (Subcutaneous plane within one thumbwidth of oral commissure)

Orbicularis oris muscle

Subcutaneous fat

Buccinator muscle

Facial artery

Mucosa

Transverse cross section view

a

Origin of superior labial artery (one thumb width from corner of mouth)

Facial artery

Inferior labial artery

Improper injection (Deep plane lateral to one thumbwidth of oral commisure)

Orbicularis oris muscle

Subcutaneous fat

Buccinator muscle

Facial artery

Mucosa

Transverse cross section view

b

Fig. 12.5 Injections in the oral commissure. **(a)** The facial artery is located one thumbwidth or 1.5 cm lateral to the oral commissure. Filler injection in the oral commissure should stay in the superficial plane within one thumbwidth from the corner of the mouth. **(b)** Injecting filler too deeply or laterally (greater than one thumbwidth from the corner of mouth) risks violating the facial artery.

12.4.2 Oral Commissure

- Inject in the superficial subcutaneous tissue (▶ **Fig. 12.5**) (**Video 12.3**).[1,2]
- Stay within a **thumbwidth** of the commissure.[1,2,6]
- Use **linear crosshatch** technique.

References

[1] Scheuer JF, III, Sieber DA, Pezeshk RA, Campbell CF, Gassman AA, Rohrich RJ. Anatomy of the Facial Danger Zones: Maximizing Safety during Soft-Tissue Filler Injections. Plast Reconstr Surg. 2017; 139(1):50e–58e

[2] Scheuer JF, III, Sieber DA, Pezeshk RA, Gassman AA, Campbell CF, Rohrich RJ. Facial Danger Zones: Techniques to Maximize Safety during Soft-Tissue Filler Injections. Plast Reconstr Surg. 2017; 139(5):1103–1108

[3] Mağden O, Edizer M, Atabey A, Tayfur V, Ergür I. Cadaveric study of the arterial anatomy of the upper lip. Plast Reconstr Surg. 2004; 114(2):355–359

[4] Tansatit T, Apinuntrum P, Phetudom T. A typical pattern of the labial arteries with implication for lip augmentation with injectable fillers. Aesthetic Plast Surg. 2014; 38(6):1083–1089

[5] Al-Hoqail RA, Meguid EM. Anatomic dissection of the arterial supply of the lips: an anatomical and analytical approach. J Craniofac Surg. 2008; 19(3):785–794

[6] Lee SH, Gil YC, Choi YJ, Tansatit T, Kim HJ, Hu KS. Topographic anatomy of the superior labial artery for dermal filler injection. Plast Reconstr Surg. 2015; 135(2):445–450

[7] Cotofana S, Pretterklieber B, Lucius R, et al. Distribution Pattern of the Superior and Inferior Labial Arteries: Impact for Safe Upper and Lower Lip Augmentation Procedures. Plast Reconstr Surg. 2017; 139(5):1075–1082

[8] Lee SH, Lee HJ, Kim YS, Kim HJ, Hu KS. What is the difference between the inferior labial artery and the horizontal labiomental artery? Surg Radiol Anat. 2015; 37(8):947–953

[9] Pinar YA, Bilge O, Govsa F. Anatomic study of the blood supply of perioral region. Clin Anat. 2005; 18(5):330–339

[10] Edizer M, Mağden O, Tayfur V, Kiray A, Ergür I, Atabey A. Arterial anatomy of the lower lip: a cadaveric study. Plast Reconstr Surg. 2003; 111(7):2176–2181

13 Facial Danger Zone 4 – Nasolabial Region

Rod J. Rohrich and Raja Mohan

Abstract

This chapter summarizes how to inject soft-tissue fillers into the nasolabial region. Patients often report a prominent nasolabial fold as they age, and one option for treatment is the injection of soft-tissue filler. The facial artery's anatomical location is intimately related to the location of the nasolabial fold. We present safe techniques for injection soft-tissue filler into this region to prevent inadvertent injury to any major facial vessels.

Keywords: filler, injectable, nasolabial fold, nasolabial region, facial artery

---

Key Points for Maximizing Filler Safety in the Nasolabial Region

- Use only FDA-approved reversible hyaluronic acid fillers in most areas of the face.
- Hyaluronic acid fillers are reversible if there is a vascular issue or problem because they can be reversed with hyaluronidase.
- In the lower two-thirds of the nasolabial fold, inject into the deep dermis or superficial subcutaneous plane just medial to the nasolabial fold (▶ **Fig. 13.1**).
- Near the alar base, inject either intradermally or in the preperiosteal plane. Use incremental deep depot injection techniques in the periapical areas (▶ **Fig. 13.1**).
- Always perform using gentle, low-pressure anterograde/retrograde injections with constant motion in 1 mL syringes.
- Do not inject along the alar rim, alar grooves, or nasal sidewall because the vasculature is superficial in these regions.

13.1 Safety Considerations in the Nasolabial Region

- When injecting the nasolabial region, knowledge of the depth and course of the facial artery is paramount to prevent complications associated with intravascular injury (▶ **Fig. 13.2**).
- In the lower two-thirds of the nasolabial fold, the facial artery course lies **beneath the muscle or in the deeper planes above the muscle** (▶ **Fig. 13.3**).
- The artery becomes **superficial** at the upper third of the nasolabial fold and is most at risk for injury at this level (▶ **Fig. 13.3**) (**Video 13.1**).
- Subcutaneous injections in the upper third of the nasolabial fold can lead to soft-tissue necrosis of the alar or malar regions if there is intravascular injury (▶ **Fig. 13.4**).
- In the upper third of the nasolabial fold and superior to it, intravascular injections into the angular artery could result in ocular embolism (▶ **Fig. 13.4**).
- The nasolabial fold is the **second most** common injection site for tissue necrosis and the third most common site leading to visual loss.[1,2]

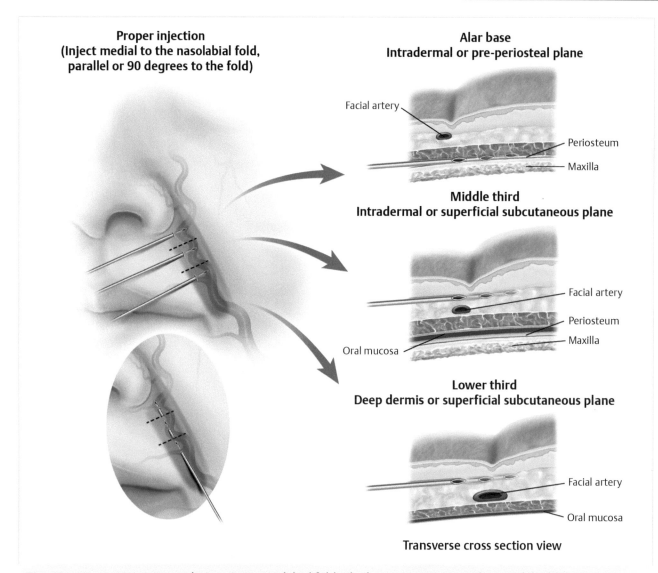

Fig. 13.1 Proper injection technique into nasolabial fold. The key in augmenting the nasolabial fold is to stay medial to the fold to prevent inadvertent injury or injections into the adjacent vasculature. In the upper third of the nasolabial zone, injections should be performed deep in a preperiosteal plane or very superficially in an intradermal plane. The artery is located within the subcutaneous tissue. In the middle third, the artery is located deeper, so injections should be performed intradermally or in a superficial subcutaneous plane. Lastly, in the lower third of the nasolabial zone, the artery is either within the muscle or between the muscle and the subcutaneous tissue, so more superficial injections are recommended.

13.2 Pertinent Anatomy of the Nasolabial Region

13.2.1 Muscles (▶ Fig. 13.2)

Orbicularis Oris

- Originates on the maxilla and mandible.
- Inserts on the skin around the perioral region.
- Function is to pucker lips.

Levator Labii Superioris

- Originates on the skin and muscle of upper lip.
- Inserts on the medial infraorbital margin.
- Elevates the upper lip.

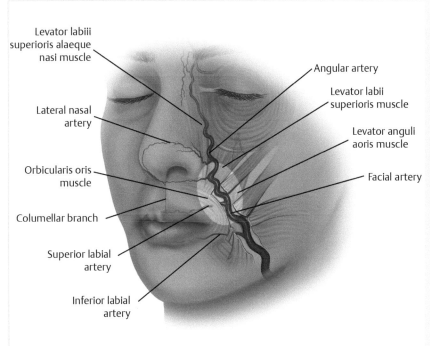

Levator labiii superioris alaeque nasi muscle

Lateral nasal artery

Orbicularis oris muscle

Columellar branch

Superior labial artery

Inferior labial artery

Angular artery

Levator labii superioris muscle

Levator anguli aoris muscle

Facial artery

Fig. 13.2 Nasolabial danger zone. The nasolabial danger zone is highlighted in the diagram. The tortuous course of the facial artery is also shown. Inferiorly, the artery is located deeper and becomes more superficial nearby the alar base. Its location is closely related to the nasolabial fold, so care must be taken when augmenting the fold. The facial artery has many important branches such as the inferior labial artery, superior labial artery, and lateral nasal artery.

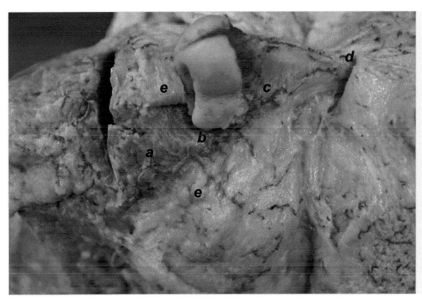

Fig. 13.3 Facial cadaver dissection highlighting details of facial artery anatomy. With the subcutaneous tissue (**e**) reflected, the facial artery (**a**) is seen running in the nasolabial fold, at times within the muscle but mostly in the plane between the subcutaneous tissue and muscle. The artery becomes superficial (**b**) in the upper third of the nasolabial fold and is at risk during superficial injections. The transition of the facial artery into the angular artery (**c**) and its anastomosis with the dorsal nasal artery (**d**) is demonstrated. Of note, the facial artery lies approximately 1.5 cm lateral to the commissure.

Levator Laii Superioris Alaeque Nasi

- Originates on the nasal bone.
- Inserts on the nostril and upper lip.
- Dilates the nostril and elevates the upper lip.

Levator Anguli Oris

- Originates on the maxilla.
- Inserts on the modiolus.
- Elevates the angle of the mouth for smiling.

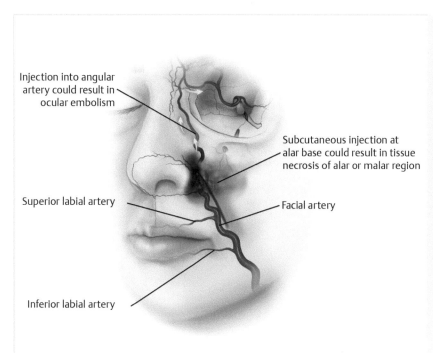

Injection into angular artery could result in ocular embolism

Subcutaneous injection at alar base could result in tissue necrosis of alar or malar region

Superior labial artery

Facial artery

Inferior labial artery

Fig. 13.4 Risk of nasolabial fold injection. Potential routes for retrograde embolization to the ophthalmic vessels are shown in the figure. Injections superficially near the alar base could result in deposits in the angular artery that can migrate in a retrograde fashion. Superficial injections near the alar base can also result in vascular compromise of the alar and malar soft tissues.

13.2.2 Vessels (▶Figs. 11.2 and ▶11.3)

Facial Artery (Video 11.1)

- The arterial portion from the cheilion (oral commissure) to the alar base is referred to as the facial artery and is adjacent to the nasolabial fold. It is approximately 1.5 cm lateral to the commissure.
- The facial artery can be medial to (42.9%), lateral to (23.2%), or across (33.9%) the nasolabial fold. [3]
- At the transition of the upper middle third and lower middle third of the nasolabial fold, the facial artery is on average 1.7 mm medial and 0.3 mm medial to the nasolabial fold at these respective sites. [3]
- The facial artery branches into the superior labial artery at the commissure and continues superiorly.
- At the ala, the facial artery becomes superficial and branches into the inferior alar artery and lateral nasal artery. [4] Beyond the ala, it is referred to as the angular artery.
- There are alternate anatomical patterns whereby an ipsilateral, duplicate facial artery may branch lower in the face and travels to the infraorbital region and cross medially to become the angular artery. [3,5,6]
- There are anatomical variations in which the angular artery is absent or arises from the ophthalmic artery. [5]
- Between the alar base and modiolus, the facial artery is either superficial to the mimetic muscles (85.2%), completely subcutaneous (16.7%), or deep to the mimetic muscles (14.8%). [7]

Superior Labial Artery

- Branch of the facial artery that follows the upper lip.
- Located between the muscle and mucosal layers.

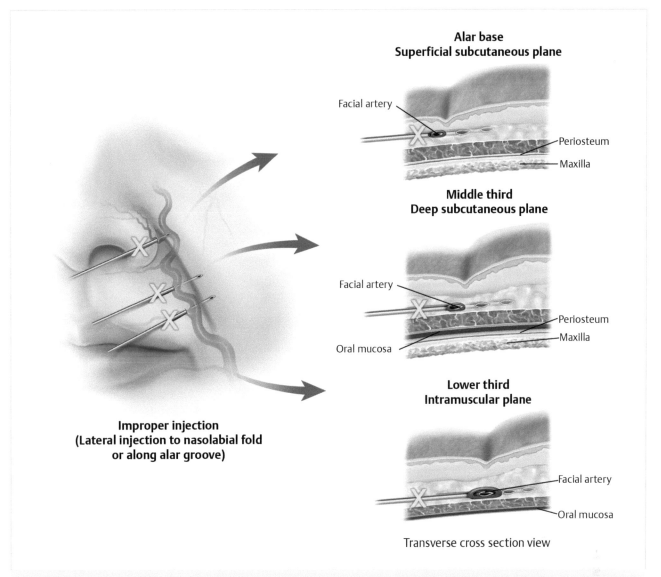

Fig. 13.5 Improper injection technique into nasolabial fold. In the upper third of the nasolabial zone, superficial injections into the subcutaneous tissue pose the greater risk of injuring the facial artery. In the middle third, deeper subcutaneous injections place the vessel at risk of injury while in the lower third, intramuscular or deeper injections can harm the facial artery. The goal is to understand the cross-sectional anatomy of the facial artery relative to the point of injection to prevent injury.

Lateral Nasal Artery

- Branch of facial artery that supplies the ala and dorsum of the nose.
- Anastomoses with the dorsal nasal branch of the ophthalmic artery.

13.3 Vascular Danger Zones and Clinical Correlations

- The facial artery in the upper third of the nasolabial fold becomes superficial, making it vulnerable to injury with relatively superficial injections (▶ **Fig. 13.5**).
- In the lower two-thirds of the nasolabial fold, inject medially to the nasolabial and laterally to the oral commissure. Inject in a superficial

plane relative to the tortuous course of the facial artery, and do not overcorrect treatment of the nasolabial fold (**Video 13.2**).

- In the upper third of the nasolabial fold starting approximately one fingerbreadth below the nasal ala, the facial artery is more superficial, so either inject in a very deep plane or use a superficial filler to address this area (**Video 13.2**).
- Use a **linear injection technique** to correct the entire nasolabial fold, and employ a **cross-radial technique** in a deeper plane for the upper third of the nasolabial fold (**Video 13.2**).
- In a fuller face, the facial artery is more lateral in the upper third of the nasolabial fold and in a face with more periapical hypoplasia, the facial artery is more medial.

References

[1] Ozturk CN, Li Y, Tung R, Parker L, Piliang MP, Zins JE. Complications following injection of soft-tissue fillers. Aesthet Surg J. 2013; 33(6):862–877

[2] Li X, Du L, Lu JJ. A Novel Hypothesis of Visual Loss Secondary to Cosmetic Facial Filler Injection. Ann Plast Surg. 2015; 75(3):258–260

[3] Yang HM, Lee JG, Hu KS, et al. New anatomical insights on the course and branching patterns of the facial artery: clinical implications of injectable treatments to the nasolabial fold and nasojugal groove. Plast Reconstr Surg. 2014; 133(5):1077–1082

[4] Nakajima H, Imanishi N, Aiso S. Facial artery in the upper lip and nose: anatomy and a clinical application. Plast Reconstr Surg. 2002; 109(3):855–861, discussion 862–863

[5] Kim YS, Choi DY, Gil YC, Hu KS, Tansatit T, Kim HJ. The anatomical origin and course of the angular artery regarding its clinical implications. Dermatol Surg. 2014; 40(10):1070–1076

[6] Niranjan NS. An anatomical study of the facial artery. Ann Plast Surg. 1988; 21(1):14–22

[7] Lee JG, Yang HM, Choi YJ, et al. Facial arterial depth and relationship with the facial musculature layer. Plast Reconstr Surg. 2015; 135(2):437–444

14 Facial Danger Zone 5 – Nasal Region

Rod J. Rohrich and Raja Mohan

Abstract

This chapter summarizes how to inject soft-tissue fillers into the nose. Many patients desire a rhinoplasty without undergoing surgery, and the concept of a "liquid rhinoplasty" involves improving the appearance of the nose using soft-tissue filler. The nasal region is highly vascular, so in this chapter we present safe techniques for injection that will avoid injury to these vascular structures. The key is to remain deep during injection.

Keywords: filler, injectable, nose, nasal region, noninvasive rhinoplasty

Key Points for Maximizing Filler Safety in the Nasal Region

- Recommend using hyaluronic acid fillers because they can be reversed with hyaluronidase. Use less hydrophilic filler to prevent delayed swelling.
- Inject small amounts with serial threading, and massage after each injection.
- Use serial puncture technique for nasal tip and ala (**Video 14.1**).
- Always inject deeply and superiorly to the alar groove for lateral injections. Never inject into the alar groove area in any layer, as this is the location of the lateral nasal artery (▶**Fig. 14.1**, ▶**Fig. 14.2**, ▶**Fig. 14.3**, ▶**Fig. 14.4**)
- In the midline, keep injections in a deep plane to avoid injury to the superficial vasculature (▶**Fig. 14.4**) (**Video 14.1**).
- The internal nasal valve can be widened with small deep injections in the midvault.
- Do not inject along the alar rim or the nasal sidewall because the vasculature is superficial in these regions (▶**Fig. 14.4**).
- Compress the dorsal nasal and angular arteries when performing injections adjacent to these blood vessels.
- Be careful in patients who have prior rhinoplasty surgery because the anatomic planes are distorted secondary to scarring.

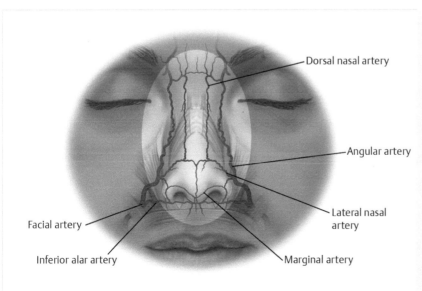

Fig. 14.1 Vasculature of the nasal aesthetic unit. The facial artery travels upward to become the angular artery. Important branches of the facial artery include the lateral nasal artery and inferior alar artery. The paired dorsal nasal arteries are located lateral to the midline along the dorsum of the nose.

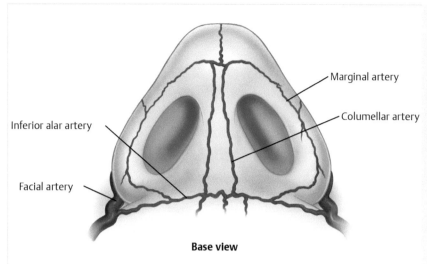

Base view

Fig. 14.2 Vasculature of the nose shown from a basal view. The inferior alar artery is a branch of the facial artery, which courses along the base of the nose. The columellar artery arises as a branch from the inferior alar artery and is divided during an open rhinoplasty. The marginal artery runs superficial along the alar rim.

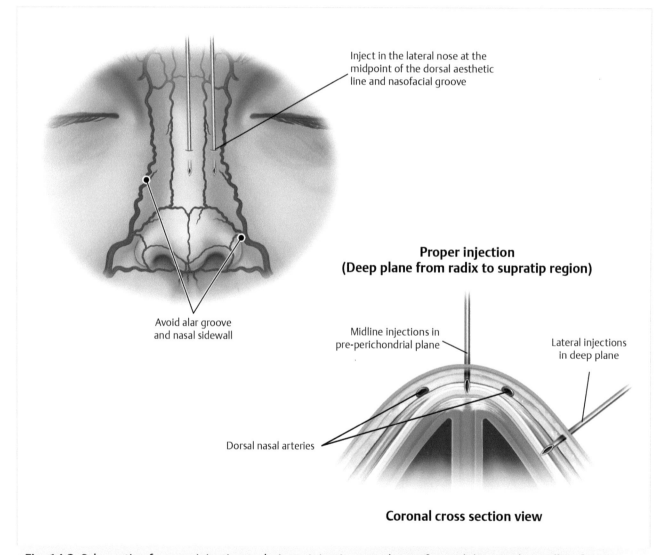

Fig. 14.3 Schematic of proper injection technique. Injections can be performed deep in the midline from the radix to the supratip break to avoid intra-vascular injection. If injections are performed laterally, they are performed deeply at the midpoint of the dorsal aesthetic line and the nasofacial groove to prevent inadvertent injury to the dorsal nasal artery and angular artery.

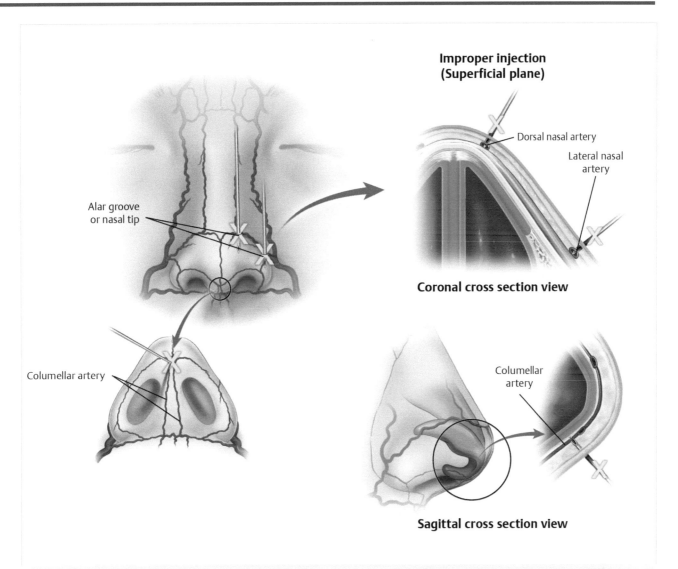

Improper injection (Superficial plane)

Dorsal nasal artery

Lateral nasal artery

Coronal cross section view

Alar groove or nasal tip

Columellar artery

Columellar artery

Sagittal cross section view

Fig. 14.4 Schematic of improper injection technique. Injections in a superficial plane lateral to the midline place the dorsal nasal artery at risk. Injections in a superficial plane along the nasal sidewall place the angular artery at risk. Injections in a superficial plane along the alar groove can compromise the lateral nasal artery. Lastly, superficial injections in the midline of the tip can injure the columellar artery.

14.1 Safety Considerations in the Nasal Region

- The layers of the nose are as follows: epidermis, dermis, subcutaneous fat, muscle, fascia, areolar tissue, perichondrium/periosteum, and cartilage/bone[1] (▶Fig. 14.5 and ▶Fig. 14.6)
- Vasculature in the nose is superficially located beneath the dermis. Injections should be carried out deep to the musculoaponeurotic layers (**Video 14.2**).
- Do not inject superficially into the alar groove or the nasal tip (▶Fig. 14.4).
- Nasal injections are the leading cause for tissue necrosis and the second most common site leading to visual loss (▶Fig. 14.7).[2,3]

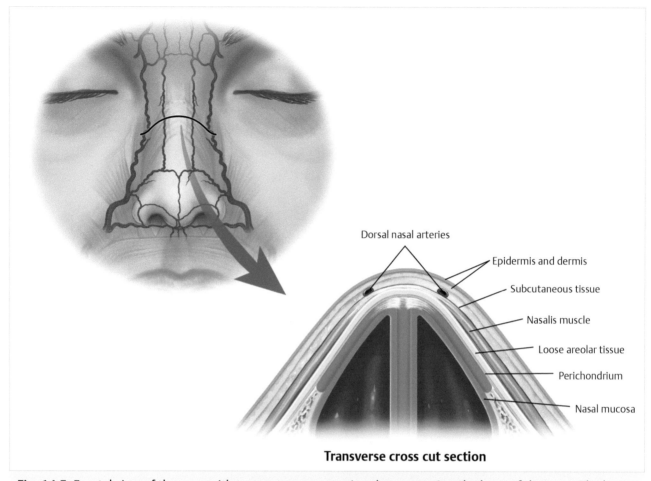

Dorsal nasal arteries
Epidermis and dermis
Subcutaneous tissue
Nasalis muscle
Loose areolar tissue
Perichondrium
Nasal mucosa

Transverse cross cut section

Fig. 14.5 Frontal view of the nose with transverse cross section demonstrating the layer of the nose. The layers of the nose (from superficial to deep) in the midvault are as follows: epidermis, dermis, subcutaneous tissue, muscle, loose areolar tissue, and perichondrium. Note that the dorsal nasal arteries are lateral to the midline, making the midline of the nose a safe place for injection, from glabella to the supratip break.

14.2 Pertinent Anatomy of the Nasal Region

14.2.1 Muscles

Nasalis

- Originates on the maxilla.
- Inserts on the nasal bone.
- The transverse portion compresses the nostrils. The alar portion dilates the nostrils.

Levator Laii Superioris Alaeque Nasi

- Originates on the nasal bone.
- Inserts on the nostril and upper lip.
- Dilates the nostril and elevates the upper lip.

Depressor Septi Nasi

- Originates on the maxilla.
- Inserts on the nasal septum.
- Depresses the nasal septum.

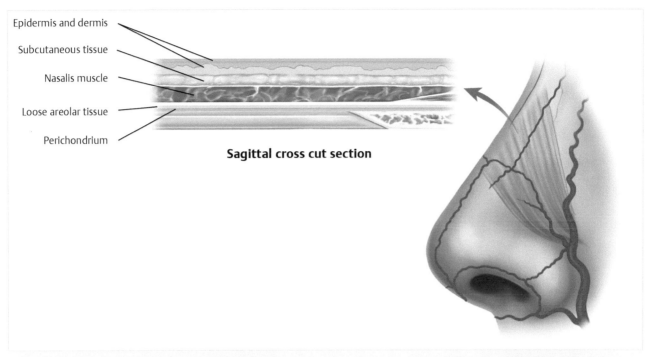

Epidermis and dermis

Subcutaneous tissue

Nasalis muscle

Loose areolar tissue

Perichondrium

Sagittal cross cut section

Fig. 14.6 Lateral view of the nose with sagittal cross section demonstrating the layers of the nose. The layers of the nose (from superficial to deep) in the midvault are as follows: epidermis, dermis, subcutaneous tissue, muscle, loose areolar tissue, and perichondrium.

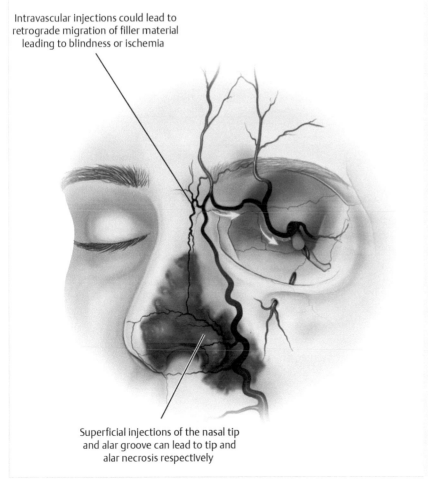

Intravascular injections could lead to retrograde migration of filler material leading to blindness or ischemia

Superficial injections of the nasal tip and alar groove can lead to tip and alar necrosis respectively

Fig. 14.7 Vascular anatomy of the periocular and nasal region. There are many potential routes for retrograde embolization to the ophthalmic vessels, including the angular and dorsal nasal arteries. Superficial injections into the nasal tip and alar groove can result in vascular compromise of the nasal tip, ala, sidewall, dorsum, and alar/cheek junction.

14.2.2 Vessels

Facial artery

- The arterial portion from the cheilion (oral commissure) to the alar base is referred to as the facial artery and is adjacent to the nasolabial fold. It is approximately 1.5 cm lateral to the commissure.
- At the ala, the facial artery becomes superficial and branches into the inferior alar artery and lateral nasal artery (▶ **Fig. 14.1** and ▶ **Fig. 14.8**).[4]

Beyond the ala, it is referred to as the angular artery and courses toward the medial canthus to anastomose with the dorsal nasal arterial system.

- The facial artery is approximately 3.2 mm lateral to the lateral-most point of the ala.[4,5]

Inferior Alar Artery and Lateral Nasal Artery

- The inferior alar artery travels along the inferior margin of the nostril, and the lateral nasal artery (**Video 14.2**) runs in the subdermal plexus superior to the alar groove over the lower lateral cartilage (▶ **Fig. 14.2**).[1,6,7,8]

Marginal Artery

- Found overlying the lower lateral cartilage and arises from the lateral nasal artery or facial artery.[8]

Dorsal Nasal Artery

- Arises from the medial orbit and travels over the dorsum to supply the nasal tip (▶ **Fig. 14.5**).[6]
- Originates from the ophthalmic artery.

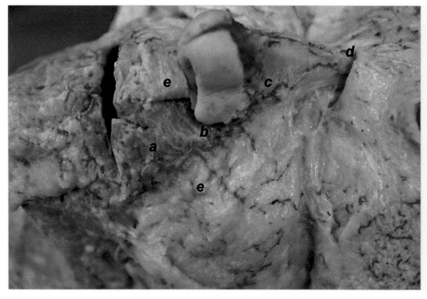

Fig. 14.8 With the subcutaneous tissue (**e**) reflected, the facial artery (**a**) is seen running in the nasolabial fold sporadically within the muscle but mostly in the plane between the subcutaneous tissue and muscle. The artery becomes superficial (**b**) in the upper third of the nasolabial fold and is at risk during superficial injections. The transition of the facial artery into the angular artery (**c**) and its anastomosis with the dorsal nasal artery (**d**) is demonstrated. Of note, the facial artery lies approximately 1.5 cm lateral to the commissure.

14.3 Vascular Danger Zones and Clinical Correlations

- The subdermal plexus is prominent in the nasal tip, and the large arterial and venous systems of the nasal skin are found superficial to the nasal musculature (superficial musculoaponeurotic system layer).[6]
- Superficial injections of the nasal tip and alar groove can lead to tip and alar necrosis, respectively (▶Fig. 14.9).
- The vasculature of the dorsum, tip, and sidewalls anastomose with the ophthalmic artery. Any intravascular injections could lead to retrograde migration of filler material which could lead to blindness or ischemia (▶Fig. 14.7).
- Lateral injections should be performed in a deep layer 3 mm superior to the alar groove.
- Midline injections into the tip and dorsum should be deep in a preperichondral or preperiosteal plane (**Video 14.1**).

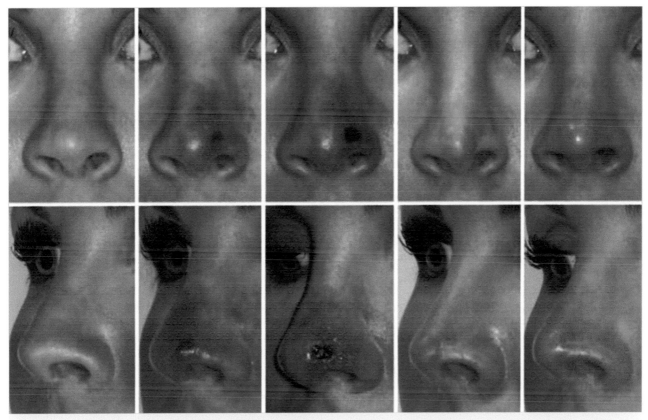

Fig. 14.9 A 36-year-old female with irregularity of right tip/alar junction and an over-reduced nasal tip after eight previous rhinoplasty operations. She was injected with 0.1 ml of Juvéderm Voluma (Allergan, Inc.) to the right tip/alar junction and 0.2 ml to the supratip and left tip/alar junction. Six days after the procedure, she began to show signs of tissue necrosis. Three separate injections delivering a total of 30 units of hyaluronidase in 1.5 ml of 2% lidocaine were injected at 10-minute intervals to the nasal tip, alae, dorsum, and sidewalls. The patient was started on 81 mg of aspirin daily, and nitropaste was applied topically every 8 hours. Hyperbaric oxygen treatment was started, and she had a total of 12 sessions. She is shown at 8 days after the procedure (*center*) with the maximum amount of tissue necrosis that she experienced. Her appearance is shown at 6 months (*second from the right*) following the initial injection and then again (*right*) after injection of 0.1 ml of Juvéderm Refine to the right tip/alar junction and 0.05 ml to the left tip/alar junction over two treatment sessions at 4-week intervals. Both the type of product and the volume injected during the session may have contributed to this complication (*Reproduced with permission from Rohrich R, Adams W, Ahmad J et al., ed. Dallas Rhinoplasty. Nasal Surgery by the Masters. 3rd Edition. Thieme; 2014*).

References

[1] Saban Y, Andretto Amodeo C, Hammou JC, Polselli R. An anatomical study of the nasal superficial musculoaponeurotic system: surgical applications in rhinoplasty. Arch Facial Plast Surg. 2008; 10(2):109–115

[2] Ozturk CN, Li Y, Tung R, Parker L, Piliang MP, Zins JE. Complications following injection of soft-tissue fillers. Aesthet Surg J. 2013; 33(6):862–877

[3] Li X, Du L, Lu JJ. A Novel Hypothesis of Visual Loss Secondary to Cosmetic Facial Filler Injection. Ann Plast Surg. 2015; 75(3):258–260

[4] Nakajima H, Imanishi N, Aiso S. Facial artery in the upper lip and nose: anatomy and a clinical application. Plast Reconstr Surg. 2002; 109(3):855–861, discussion 862–863

[5] Yang HM, Lee JG, Hu KS, et al. New anatomical insights on the course and branching patterns of the facial artery: clinical implications of injectable treatments to the nasolabial fold and nasojugal groove. Plast Reconstr Surg. 2014; 133(5):1077–1082

[6] Toriumi DM, Mueller RA, Grosch T, Bhattacharyya TK, Larrabee WF, Jr. Vascular anatomy of the nose and the external rhinoplasty approach. Arch Otolaryngol Head Neck Surg. 1996; 122(1):24–34

[7] Rohrich RJ, Gunter JP, Friedman RM. Nasal tip blood supply: an anatomic study validating the safety of the transcolumellar incision in rhinoplasty. Plast Reconstr Surg. 1995; 95(5):795–799, discussion 800–801

[8] Saban Y, Andretto Amodeo C, Bouaziz D, Polselli R. Nasal arterial vasculature: medical and surgical applications. Arch Facial Plast Surg. 2012; 14(6):429–436

15 Facial Danger Zone 6 – Infraorbital Region

Rod J. Rohrich and Raja Mohan

Abstract

This chapter summarizes how to inject soft-tissue fillers into the infraorbital region. Patients often report hollowness in their lower eyelid consistent with a tear trough deformity. To blend the lid/cheek junction, we present techniques to safely augment the lower eyelid and cheek. The infraorbital nerve and artery are located within the infraorbital region, and detailed knowledge of the anatomy is key to prevent devastating complications such as blindness.

Keywords: filler, injectable, periorbital region, tear trough, infraorbital region

---

Key Points for Maximizing Filler Safety in the Infraorbital Region

- Use low-G' fillers and less hydrophilic fillers.
- It it better to use hyaluronic acid fillers because they can be reversed with hyaluronidase. This is especially important in the tear trough.
- Inject small amounts in a low-pressure manner, always doing so in a retrograde and anterograde manner.
- Avoid direct, deep injections into the location of the infraorbital foramen (▶ Fig. 15.1 and ▶ Fig. 15.2). Best practice is to inject inferiorly and laterally to the location of the foramen.
- The primary injection sites for blending follow the zygomatic arch and are along the malar eminence (▶ Fig. 15.3). Secondary injection sites are below the zygomatic arch, inframalar region, and the superficial fat compartments of the midface (**Video 15.1**).
- Inject the lateral two-thirds of the tear trough from a lateral direction and stay in a deep (preperiosteal) plane (▶ Fig. 15.4).
- Inject the medial one-third of the tear trough from an inferior direction, staying in a deep plane. Inject a low volume in a cross-hatching pattern (**Video 15.1**).

15.1 Safety Considerations in the Infraorbital Region

- When injecting the infraorbital region, knowledge of the depth of injection and anatomy of the region is needed to prevent vascular injury (▶ Fig. 15.1,▶ Fig. 15.2).
- Cannulation of the infraorbital artery and injection of filler could lead to devastating complications of blindness with retrograde migration of filler (▶ Fig. 15.6).
- Insult to the infraorbital nerve can lead to sensory changes and pain.
- Assess the malar highlights and the tear trough to determine where the patient will benefit most from injectable filler. The key is to subtly enhance the area without adding too much volume.

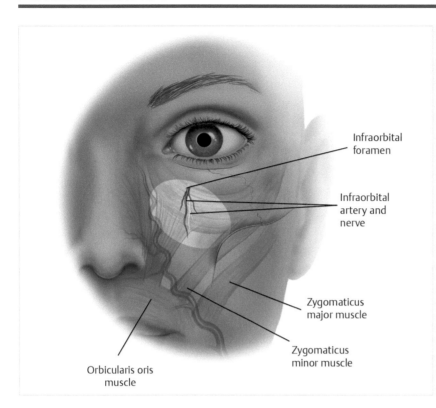

Fig. 15.1 Anatomy of the Periocular Region. The infraorbital artery and nerve emanate from the infraorbital foramen.

Infraorbital foramen

Infraorbital artery and nerve

Zygomaticus major muscle

Zygomaticus minor muscle

Orbicularis oris muscle

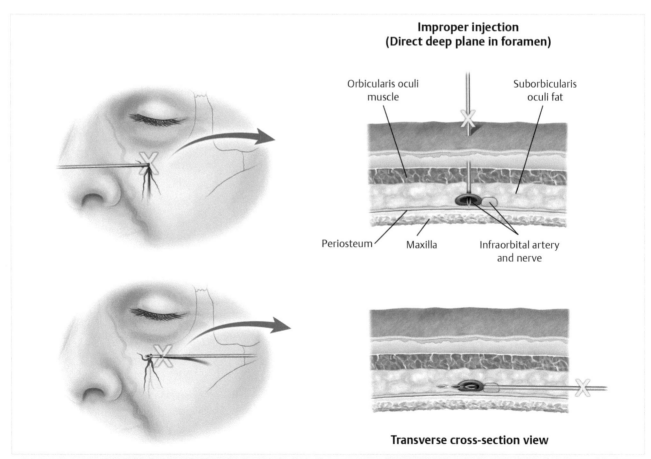

Improper injection
(Direct deep plane in foramen)

Orbicularis oculi muscle

Suborbicularis oculi fat

Periosteum   Maxilla   Infraorbital artery and nerve

Transverse cross-section view

Fig. 15.2 Improper Injection Technique. Direct injections overlying the infraorbital foramen should not be performed. Furthermore, lateral injections should not deposit filler near the infraorbital foramen. One should be very cautious when filling the tear trough and not deposit filler near it. Intravascular injections can result in migration of emboli in a retrograde fashion to the ophthalmic artery.

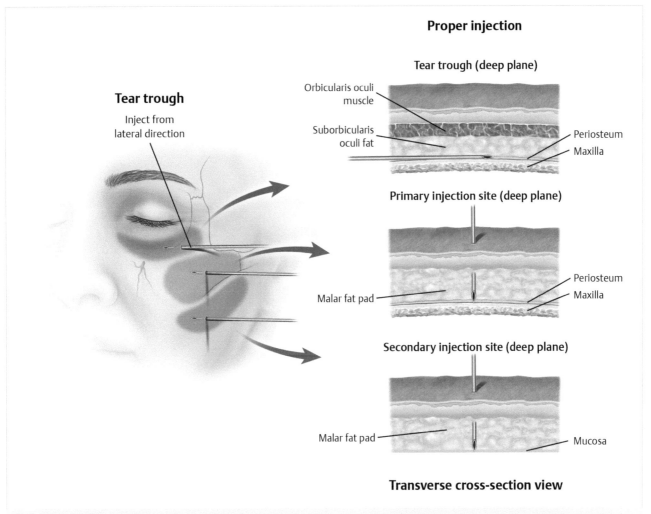

Proper injection

Tear trough (deep plane)

Orbicularis oculi muscle

Suborbicularis oculi fat

Periosteum

Maxilla

Tear trough

Inject from lateral direction

Primary injection site (deep plane)

Malar fat pad

Periosteum

Maxilla

Secondary injection site (deep plane)

Malar fat pad

Mucosa

Transverse cross-section view

Fig. 15.3 Tear Trough and Malar Eminence Injection Technique. When injecting from the tear trough laterally, the needle should be in a deep preperiosteal plane. Injections should not be performed adjacent to the infraorbital foramen. The malar and zygomatic eminence can be filled laterally by performing depot injections in a deep plane. The needle should be perpendicular to the skin surface for these volumizing injections.

15.2 Pertinent Anatomy of the Infraorbital Region

15.2.1 Muscles (▶Fig. 15.1)

Orbicularis Oris

- Originates on the maxilla and mandible.
- Inserts on the skin around perioral region.
- Function is to pucker the lips.

Zygomaticus Major

- Originates on the zygomatic bone.
- Inserts on the modiolus.
- Elevates the upper lip and angle of the mouth.

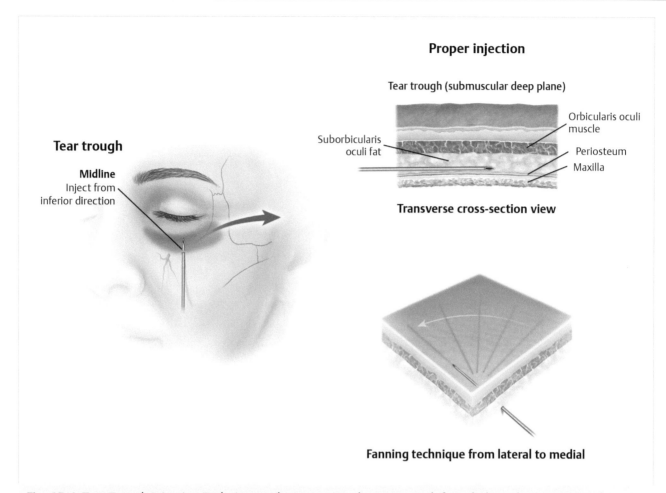

Proper injection

Tear trough (submuscular deep plane)

Suborbicularis oculi fat

Orbicularis oculi muscle

Periosteum

Maxilla

Transverse cross-section view

Tear trough

Midline
Inject from
inferior direction

Fanning technique from lateral to medial

Fig. 15.4 Tear Trough Injection Technique. When injecting the tear trough from below, the trajectory of the needle should be lateral to the location of the infraorbital foramen. The needle should be in a deep preperiosteal plane, and the needle can be fanned laterally to add more volume. Injections should not be performed near the infraorbital foramen.

Zygomaticus Minor

- Originates on the zygoma.
- Inserts on the upper lip.
- Elevates the upper lip.

15.2.2 Vessels

Infraorbital Artery/Nerve

- The infraorbital foramen is located approximately 6.3 to 10.9 mm below the infraorbital rim (▶ **Fig. 15.5**). This distance corresponds to approximately 33 to 41% of the distance between the canthi[1,2,3,4,5,6,7] (**Video 15.2**).
- The foramen is approximately 25.7 to 27.1 mm from the midline in men and 24.2 to 26.8 mm in women.[2,3,4,5,6]
- 30% of the time, the infraorbital foramen is in the same vertical plane as the supraorbital foramen.[2]
- The foramen is also in line with the following teeth: premolar, second premolar, canines.[2,3]
- Some patients have multiple foramina.[1,4,8]

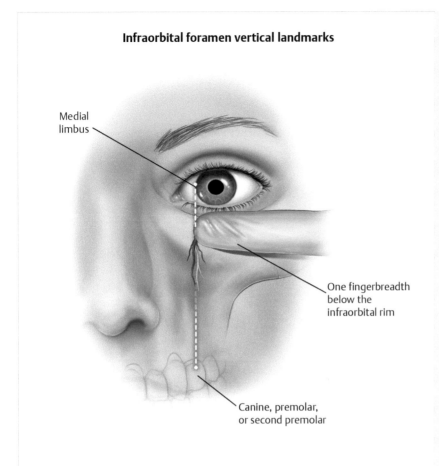

Infraorbital foramen vertical landmarks

Medial limbus

One fingerbreadth below the infraorbital rim

Canine, premolar, or second premolar

Fig. 15.5 Infraorbital foramen. The foramen is located approximately one fingerbreadth below the infraorbital rim. A vertical line drawn from the medial limbus helps determine its location. When filling the tear trough or the malar eminence, one should be cautious and keep in mind where the infraorbital foramen is located.

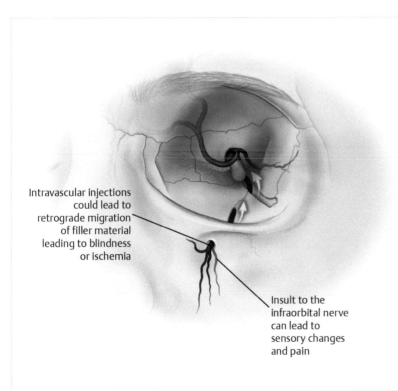

Intravascular injections could lead to retrograde migration of filler material leading to blindness or ischemia

Insult to the infraorbital nerve can lead to sensory changes and pain

Fig. 15.6 Potential routes for retrograde embolization to the ophthalmic vessels. Intravascular injections into the infraorbital artery can migrate in a retrograde fashion and lead to blindness or ischemia. Pressure or injury to the infraorbital nerve can induce paresthesia and numbness.

15.3 Vascular Danger Zones and Clinical Correlations

- The infraorbital foramen is in line with the medial limbus in a vertical plane. It is approximately one fingerbreadth below the infraorbital rim (▶**Fig. 15.5**).
- Keep the anatomical measurements in mind when injecting the infraorbital region.
- Injections in the infraorbital region should be lateral to the location of the infraorbital foramen.
- Injections medial to the location of the infraorbital region should be approached with caution. Filler in this area can be added deep and pushed medially if needed.
- The facial vein is lateral to the infraorbital foramen and located more superficially. Avoid injection into this vein by staying deep in it (**Video 15.2**).

References

[1] Canan S, Asim OM, Okan B, Ozek C, Alper M. Anatomic variations of the infraorbital foramen. Ann Plast Surg. 1999; 43(6):613–617

[2] Aziz SR, Marchena JM, Puran A. Anatomic characteristics of the infraorbital foramen: a cadaver study. J Oral Maxillofac Surg. 2000; 58(9):992–996

[3] Raschke R, Hazani R, Yaremchuk MJ. Identifying a safe zone for midface augmentation using anatomic landmarks for the infraorbital foramen. Aesthet Surg J. 2013; 33(1):13–18

[4] Aggarwal A, Kaur H, Gupta T, et al. Anatomical study of the infraorbital foramen: A basis for successful infraorbital nerve block. Clin Anat. 2015; 28(6):753–760

[5] Cutright B, Quillopa N, Schubert W. An anthropometric analysis of the key foramina for maxillofacial surgery. J Oral Maxillofac Surg. 2003; 61(3):354–357

[6] Hwang SH, Kim SW, Park CS, Kim SW, Cho JH, Kang JM. Morphometric analysis of the infraorbital groove, canal, and foramen on three-dimensional reconstruction of computed tomography scans. Surg Radiol Anat. 2013; 35(7):565–571

[7] Liu DN, Guo JL, Luo Q, et al. Location of supraorbital foramen/notch and infraorbital foramen with reference to soft- and hard-tissue landmarks. J Craniofac Surg. 2011; 22(1):293–296

[8] Agthong S, Huanmanop T, Chentanez V. Anatomical variations of the supraorbital, infraorbital, and mental foramina related to gender and side. J Oral Maxillofac Surg. 2005; 63(6):800–804

Part III

Energy-Based Devices

Erez Dayan, Rod J. Rohrich,
E. Victor Ross

16 Maximizing Safety with Ablative Lasers

E. Victor Ross, Erez Dayan, and Rod J. Rohrich

Abstract

Lasers are among the most precise and powerful tools available in facial rejuvenation. Through selective photothermolysis, lasers are able to target specific tissue chromophores based on their absorption wavelength (i.e., hemoglobin, water, melanin). Laser technology and safety have evolved significantly since the continuous wave CO_2 laser developed in 1964, which had less control of energy parameters, leading to frequent injury and scarring. The pulsed mode (and subsequent superpulse and ultrapulse lasers) was a significant advance in safety and efficacy. This technology uses electronic shutters to interrupt the continuous wave of energy into pulses, thereby limiting thermal damage. The introduction of the Er:YAG laser in the mid-1990s offered a more selective absorption of water (12–18 x) than CO_2 lasers with less collateral heat injury to surrounding tissues.

Perhaps the most significant modern advance in the safety and efficacy of lasers was the evolution of the fractional laser in 2003. Fractional thermolysis resurfaces microtreatment zones (MTZ) within a target area (typically 20%); maintaining intervening uninjured epidermis and dermis that preserves the skin's barrier function while speeding re-epithelialization.

Keywords: laser, selective photothermolysis, laser resurfacing, ablation, skin resurfacing, fractional laser, CO2 laser, Er, YAG laser

---

Key Points

- The most common ablative lasers used in facial aesthetics are CO_2 and Er:YAG. Both target water as a chromophore. Er:YAG is more specific (12–18 x), leading to less surrounding heat dissipation and collateral tissue damage.[1,2,3,4,5]
- The goal of ablative lasers is to eliminate or reduce damaged collagen and encourage new collagen formation and remodeling through a combination of tissue vaporization and collagen denaturation secondary to thermal damage.[6,7,8]
- Ablative fractional lasers lead to microthermal zones of injury, with surrounding areas reaching temperatures of 55–62°C. This denatures existing collagen, leading to neocollagenesis, elastogenesis, and remodeling.[1,9,10,11]
- Ablative lasers can be used on patients of all skin types; however, to avoid permanent hypo or hyperpigmentation and scarring, treatment should be avoided or approached with extreme caution in patients with > Fitzpatrick type III skin.[9,10]

16.1 Safety Considerations

- CO_2 Laser (10,600 nm)
- CO_2 lasers have a higher ablation threshold than Erbium lasers, which means that greater thermal heating is required to achieve effect.[9,10]
- Ablation is achieved at 5 J/cm² for CO_2 lasers with a residual 70–150 μm area of heating.[9,10]

- Depth of ablation depends on the number of passes, the fluence, the pulse duration, and the amount of cooling time between passes.[1,11]
- As more passes of the CO_2 laser are performed, less water (target chromophore) is present to be vaporized. This leads to additive heat accumulation and increased potential for thermal injury/scarring.
- Clinical endpoint depends on color assessment of tissue (as in chemical peels) rather than dermal bleeding.[1,6,11,12]
- Fractional CO_2 lasers allow for the creation of microthermal zones (MTZ) of pixilated tissue damage to the underlying dermis while leaving epidermal elements intact. This allows for more rapid re-epithelialization and dermal collagen remodeling. Thus, multiple treatments can be achieved with less risk for pigmentation changes. Coverage density ranges from 10 to 60% per pass depending on the area being treated.[3]

16.2 Er:YAG Laser (2950 nm)

- The Er:YAG laser has the same chromophore as CO_2 laser (water) but is more specific, leading to less thermal diffusion and theoretically increased safety.[13,14]
- Ablation is achieved at 0.5 J/cm² for Erbium lasers with a 5–20 μm area of residual heating.[13,14]
- Due to less generation of heat compared to CO_2 laser, the Erbium laser does not have the same effect on collagen remodeling/deposition and is not as effective for skin tightening.[2,13,15]
- Erbium lasers have less depth of penetration compared to CO_2 lasers and are often used to treat more superficial areas (i.e., epidermal lesions, actinic damage, dyspigmentation). However, with higher fluence in multiple passes, they can achieve very deep resurfacing depths and cause scarring.
- Clinical endpoint is punctate papillary dermal bleeding and fragmented appearance of dermis. With this particular laser, pulse durations are increased and significant coagulation can be achieved similar to what is typically observed with the CO_2 laser.

16.3 Pertinent Anatomy

- Safe zones for ablative laser resurfacing (fractional or continuous) include areas with thicker dermis and ample perfusion, including central cheeks, forehead, and nose (▶ Fig. 16.1). Multiple passes may be applied in these areas to achieve optimal results.
- Danger zones include areas with thinner dermis or areas that may have been undermined during surgery (i.e., in a facelift/necklift) and include: neck, upper chest, eyelids, and periorbital areas (▶ Fig. 16.1)

16.4 Technical Points

- In areas that have thinner dermis or have been undermined, the laser is obliquely oriented to decrease the degree of ablation (▶ Fig. 16.2). Settings may also be decreased in these areas (by 30–50%) to avoid bulk heating and scarring.

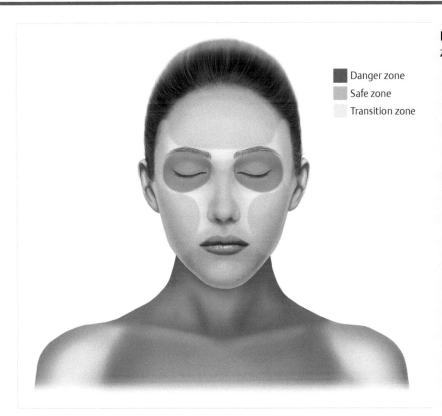

Fig. 16.1 Safe zones and danger zones for ablative laser resurfacing.

Danger zone
Safe zone
Transition zone

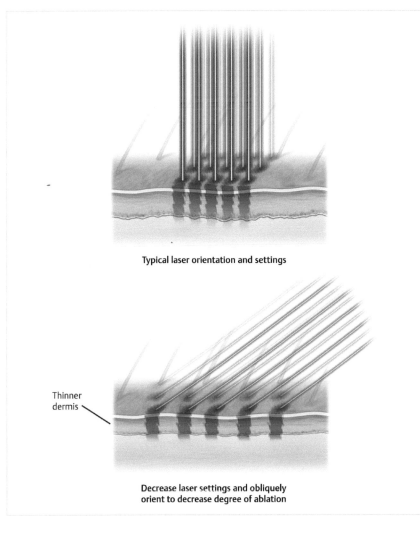

Typical laser orientation and settings

Thinner dermis

Decrease laser settings and obliquely orient to decrease degree of ablation

Fig. 16.2 Technique to maximize safety when performing laser after facelift/necklift.

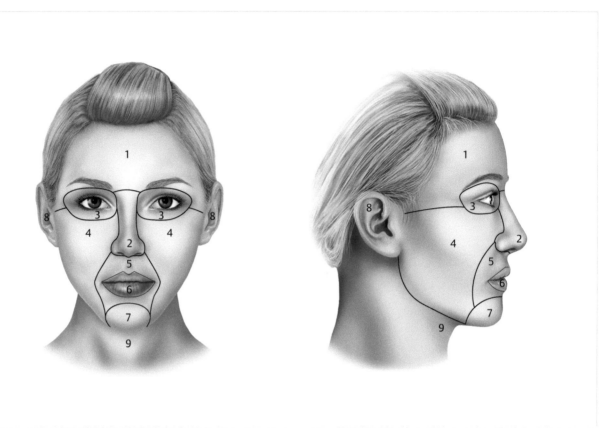

Fig. 16.3 Aesthetic units of the face.

- Aesthetic units are treated and blended with each other to avoid noticeable transition points (▸**Fig. 16.3**).
- The treated areas are assessed continuously until tissue turns white/yellow (CO_2) or petechial papillary dermal bleeding is encountered (Er:YAG) as a clinical endpoint.
- Spot treatment can be utilized to treat peeks of deeper rhytids (typically in the perioral region).

References

[1] Duplechain JK, Rubin MG, Kim K. Novel post-treatment care after ablative and fractional CO2 laser resurfacing. J Cosmet Laser Ther. 2014; 16(2):77–82

[2] El-Domyati M, Abd-El-Raheem T, Abdel-Wahab H, et al. Fractional versus ablative erbium: yttrium-aluminum-garnet laser resurfacing for facial rejuvenation: an objective evaluation. J Am Acad Dermatol. 2013; 68(1):103–112

[3] Griffin D, Brelsford M, O'Reilly E, Stroup SP, Shumaker P. Ablative Fractional Laser Resurfacing: A Promising Adjunct to Surgical Reconstruction. Mil Med. 2016; 181(6):e616–e620

[4] Burns C, Basnett A, Valentine J, Shumaker P. Ablative fractional laser resurfacing: A powerful tool to help restore form and function during international medical exchange. Lasers Surg Med. 2017; 49(5):471–474

[5] Hassan KM, Benedetto AV. Facial skin rejuvenation: ablative laser resurfacing, chemical peels, or photodynamic therapy? Facts and controversies. Clin Dermatol. 2013; 31(6):737–740

[6] Clementoni MT, Lavagno R, Munavalli G. A new multi-modal fractional ablative CO2 laser for wrinkle reduction and skin resurfacing. J Cosmet Laser Ther. 2012; 14(6):244–252

[7] Çalıskan E, Açıkgöz G, Tunca M, Koç E, Arca E, Akar A. Treatment of lipoid proteinosis with ablative Er:YAG laser resurfacing. Dermatol Ther (Heidelb). 2015; 28(5):291–295

[8] Cohen JL, Ross EV. Combined fractional ablative and nonablative laser resurfacing treatment: a split-face comparative study. J Drugs Dermatol. 2013; 12(2):175–178

[9] Rohrich RJ, Gyimesi IM, Clark P, Burns AJ. CO_2 laser safety considerations in facial skin resurfacing. Plast Reconstr Surg. 1997; 100(5):1285–1290

[10] Schwartz RJ, Burns AJ, Rohrich RJ, Barton FE, Jr, Byrd HS. Long-term assessment of CO_2 facial laser resurfacing: aesthetic results and complications. Plast Reconstr Surg. 1999; 103(2):592–601

[11] Tierney EP, Hanke CW, Petersen J. Ablative fractionated CO_2 laser treatment of photoaging: a clinical and histologic study. Dermatol Surg. 2012; 38(11):1777–1789

[12] Cartee TV, Wasserman DI. Commentary: Ablative fractionated CO2 laser treatment of photoaging: a clinical and histologic study. Dermatol Surg. 2012; 38(11):1790–1793

[13] Farshidi D, Hovenic W, Zachary C. Erbium:yttrium aluminum garnet ablative laser resurfacing for skin tightening. Dermatol Surg. 2014; 40(Suppl 12):S152–S156

[14] Lee SJ, Kang JM, Chung WS, Kim YK, Kim HS. Ablative non-fractional lasers for atrophic facial acne scars: a new modality of erbium:YAG laser resurfacing in Asians. Lasers Med Sci. 2014; 29(2):615–619

[15] Tao J, Champlain A, Weddington C, Moy L, Tung R. Treatment of burn scars in Fitzpatrick phototype III patients with a combination of pulsed dye laser and non-ablative fractional resurfacing 1550 nm erbium:glass/1927 nm thulium laser devices. Scars Burn Heal. 2018; 4:2059513118758510

17 Maximizing Safety with Nonablative Lasers

E. Victor Ross, Erez Dayan, and Rod J. Rohrich

Abstract

Nonablative lasers are commonly used to treat a variety of conditions such as dyschromia, fine rhytids, acne scars, tattoos, burn scars, hair removal, and striae. Through selective photothermolysis, lasers are able to target specific tissue chromophores based on their absorption wavelength (i.e., hemoglobin, water, melanin) while being minimally absorbed by adjacent nontarget tissue. The goal of nonablative laser resurfacing, and its primary difference compared to ablative lasers, is to restore damaged collagen without injuring or removing the overlaying epidermis. Nonablative lasers typically lead to less downtime compared to ablative laser treatments but are also associated with less dramatic results.

Keywords: laser, selective photothermolysis, laser resurfacing, nonablative laser, mid-infrared lasers, Nd, YAG laser, Q-Switched Nd, YAG laser, Diode laser, Fraxel, tattoo removal, hair reduction

Key Points

- The most common nonablative lasers used in facial aesthetics include: Nd:YAG, Q-switched Nd:YAG, Diode, Erbium glass fractional, visible light, and intense pulsed light devices.[1,2,3,4]
- Nonablative lasers are variably and moderately effective at reducing fine rhytids. Deeper rhytids are difficult to improve, and may require ablative lasers, chemical peel, and/or soft-tissue fillers.[3,5,6]

17.1 Safety Considerations

- Wavelength-specific safety equipment (i.e., eye protection) is required. When performed in the operating room, a laser-safe endotracheal tube must be used, and the lowest possible FiO2 should be given. Wet towels are applied around the treatment area to absorb heat energy and reduce risk of fire.[4,7]
- A test area can be used to identify the optimal fluence for the patient's skin.
- There are usually no visual endpoints for nonablative lasers used for the treatment of rhytids.[8,9,10]
- For hypervascular lesions, the treatment endpoint is mild purpura, persistent bluing of the vessels, or stenosis of the vessels.[1,7]
- For tattoo removal, the treatment endpoint is skin whitening.[11]
- Hypopigmentation (10–20%) is thought to be caused by melanocyte destruction secondary to heat injury. This is often transient and self-limited. Rarely delayed hypopigmentation can present 6–12 months after treatment.[1]
- Scarring is rare with nonablative lasers. Blistering may occur and is typically treated with antibiotic ointment until healed.[3,4,7,10]

17.2 Clinical Correlations

- Scars: combination treatments of different nonablative lasers may be most effective. For example, fractional lasers improve scar pliability, while pulsed dye laser (PDL) or intense pulse light (IPL) serve to improve erythema, hypervascularity, and dyschromia.
- Dyschromia: lentigines are treated with lasers that target melanin as chromophore.Such lasers include Q-switched lasers such as the 532 nm laser, the ruby laser, and the 755 nm alexandrite laser. Longer pulsed technologies include a wide range of visible light devices, from the long-pulse 532 nm KTP laser to the pulse dye laser and finally IPL.
- Hypervascularity: PDL, 532 nm KTP laser, and IPL are all effective. PDL can be used with purpuric and nonpurpuric settings.
- Tattoo removal: Nonablative lasers break up large particles into smaller particles to be phagocytosed by macrophages. The ideal laser depends on tattoo color, but Q-switched lasers are ideal for tattoo removal. Patients must be aware that multiple treatments may be required (as many as 10–15 in some cases).
- Hair reduction: lasers target melanin in the dermal papilla to destroy the hair follicle. Typically, lasers used include 810 diode, 755 alexandrite, and 1064 Nd:YAG. IPL is also effective for many patients. Laser hair reduction is most effective in patients with light skin and dark hair.

References

[1] Ang P, Barlow RJ. Nonablative laser resurfacing: a systematic review of the literature. Clin Exp Dermatol. 2002; 27(8):630–635

[2] Goldberg DJ. Nonablative laser technology Radiofrequency. Aesthet Surg J. 2004; 24(2):180–181

[3] Hardaway CA, Ross EV. Nonablative laser skin remodeling. Dermatol Clin. 2002; 20(1): 97–111, ix

[4] Pozner JN, Goldberg DJ. Nonablative laser resurfacing: state of the art 2002. Aesthet Surg J. 2002; 22(5):427–434

[5] Doshi SN, Alster TS. 1,450 nm long-pulsed diode laser for nonablative skin rejuvenation. Dermatol Surg. 2005; 31(9 Pt 2):1223–1226, discussion 1226

[6] Karmisholt KE, Banzhaf CA, Glud M, et al. Laser treatments in early wound healing improve scar appearance: a randomized split-wound trial with nonablative fractional laser exposures vs. untreated controls. Br J Dermatol. 2018; 179(6):1307–1314

[7] Narurkar VA. Nonablative fractional laser resurfacing. Dermatol Clin. 2009; 27(4): 473–478, vi

[8] Ross EV. Nonablative laser rejuvenation in men. Dermatol Ther. 2007; 20(6):414–429

[9] Weiss RA, McDaniel DH, Geronemus RG. Review of nonablative photorejuvenation: reversal of the aging effects of the sun and environmental damage using laser and light sources. Semin Cutan Med Surg. 2003; 22(2):93–106

[10] Williams EF, III, Dahiya R. Review of nonablative laser resurfacing modalities. Facial Plast Surg Clin North Am. 2004; 12(3):305–310, v

[11] Naga LI, Alster TS. Laser Tattoo Removal: An Update. Am J Clin Dermatol. 2017; 18(1):59–65

18 Trichloroacetic Acid Combined with Jessner's Chemical Peel Safety

Erez Dayan and Rod J. Rohrich

Abstract

Trichloroacetic acid (TCA) is a versatile agent, efficacious in treating a spectrum of facial rhytids at varying concentrations. TCA is commonly used in a 30 to 35% concentration to achieve a medium-depth peel into the upper reticular dermis. The addition of Jessner's solution prior to the TCA peel application leads to partial removal of the epidermis, allowing for deeper penetration of the TCA. This combination is beneficial, as lower concentrations of TCA can be used for the same depth of peel, minimizing complications such as scarring.

Keywords: trichloroacetic acid, TCA, chemical peel, facial rejuvenation, skin resurfacing

---

Key Points for Maximizing Chemical Peel Safety

- The type of chemical peel selected is based on the depth of penetration required to effectively treat a given condition as well as the skin type and skin thickness. As such, chemical peels are frequently classified based on depth of penetration (superficial, medium, and deep) (▶ Table 18.1).
- TCA is commonly used in a 30 to 35% concentration to achieve a medium-depth peel into the upper reticular dermis.
- A number of factors other than the concentration of TCA contributes to the depth of peel obtained, such as skin preparation, pretreatment skin type, and method of application.

▶ Table 18.1 Types of chemical peels and depth of penetration

	Depth of penetration	Peeling agent	Conditions
Superficial	Stratum corneum to papillary dermis (60 μm)	• Alpha hydroxyl acids • Beta hydroxyl acids • Jessner solution	• Mild photoaging • Mild acne scarring • Pigmentary disorders
Medium	Papillary dermis to upper reticular dermis (450 μm)	• TCA 35–50% • TCA 35% + glycolic acid 70% • TCA 35% + Jessner's solution	• Mild-to-moderate photoaging • Actinic keratosis • Fine rhytids • Solar lentigines • Pigmentary disorders
Deep	Mid-reticular dermis to 600 μm	• Baker-Gordon • TCA > 50%	• Severe photoaging • Pigmentary disorders • Premalignant skin tumors • scars

18.1 Safety Considerations

- A careful history and physical examination allows for the clinician to determine the patient's candidacy (▶Table 18.2).
- The senior author's (R.J.R.) preference is to pretreat all patients for 4 to 6 weeks prior to chemical peeling.[1,2] This regimen includes topical tretinoin (0.05–0.1%), hydroquinone (2–4%), sunscreen, and alpha hydroxyl acid (4–10%). Pretreatment improves skin tolerance, regulates fibroblast and melanocyte function, improves dermal circulation, and allows for the treated skin to heal 3 to 4 days faster due to increased cellular division and new collagen formation.[1,3,4]
- Safety and consistency are prioritized to ensure optimal results. In the case of 35% TCA peel combined with Jessner's solution, this begins with a set-up of four clearly labeled glasses ordered from left to right in the appropriate sequence of usage.
- The glasses are filled by the operating surgeon with:
  1. 70% ethyl alcohol (cleanser).
  2. acetone (degreasing agent).
  3. Jessner's solution (provides a uniform superficial exfoliation).
  4. 35% TCA acid solution.[1]

- The addition of Jessner's solution prior to TCA peel application leads to partial removal of the epidermis, allowing for deeper penetration of the TCA. This combination is beneficial, as lower concentrations of TCA can be used for the same depth of peel, minimizing complications such as scarring.[4]
- All patients are given 24 hours of prophylactic antibiotics. Acyclovir is initiated 2 days prior to chemical peel and continued 5 days after the peel in patients with a prior history of herpetic lesions.

18.2 Danger Zones and Clinical Correlations

- Safe zones include areas with thicker dermis and ample perfusion, including the central cheeks, forehead, and nose. Multiple passes of TCA may be applied to achieve optimal results (▶Fig. 18.1).
- Danger zones include areas with thinner dermis or areas that may have been undermined during surgery (i.e., a facelift or necklift) and include the neck, upper chest, eyelids, and periorbital areas. Caution should be exercised to control depth of peel in these regions.

▶ Table 18.2 Indications and contraindications of chemical peel

Indications for chemical peel	Contraindications
Superficial or deep rhytids/photoaging	Isoretinoin therapy within the previous 6 months
Preneoplastic or neoplastic lesions (i.e., actinic keratosis and lentigines)	Absence of pilosebaceous units on the face
Underlying skin disease (i.e., acne)	Infection or open wounds (herpes, open acne cysts)
Pigmentary dyschromias	Medium or deep resurfacing procedure within 3–12 months*
	Recent facial surgery involving undermining*
	History of therapeutic radiation exposure
	Fitzpatrick skin types IV, V, and VI*

*Relative contraindication

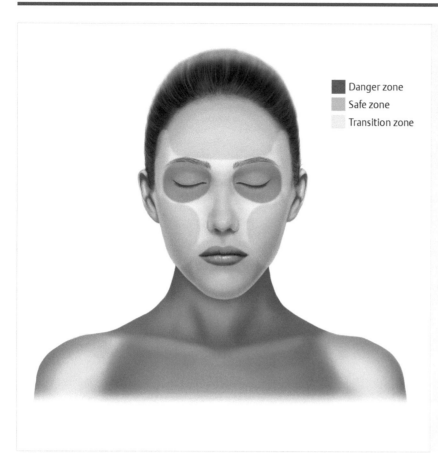

Fig. 18.1 Safe zones for chemical peel (*green*) are areas with thicker dermis. Caution must be exercise in transition (*yellow*) and danger zones (*red*) which have thinner dermis.

Danger zone
Safe zone
Transition zone

18.3 Technical Points

- We use a three-finger technique to allow for a wide and consistent surface area to be covered (Video 18.1).[4]
- A cotton-tip applicator wrung with TCA is used to treat rhytids in the periorbital and perioral region. The skin in these areas is stretched to allow for the peel to reach the bottom of the rhytids. The wooden end of the cotton tip applicator can be used for selective application of the peel for deeper rhytids.[1]
- The margin of the area being peeled (typically the mandibular border for facial peel) is lightly feathered to allow for a natural and inconspicuous transition. These areas are all constantly reassessed for color changes to assess depth and efficacy of the peel.

References

[1] Herbig K, Trussler AP, Khosla RK, Rohrich RJ. Combination Jessner's solution and trichloroacetic acid chemical peel: technique and outcomes. Plast Reconstr Surg. 2009; 124(3): 955–964

[2] Pannucci CJ, Reavey PL, Kaweski S, et al. A randomized controlled trial of skin care protocols for facial resurfacing: lessons learned from the Plastic Surgery Educational Foundation's Skin Products Assessment Research study. Plast Reconstr Surg. 2011; 127(3):1334–1342

[3] Johnson JB, Ichinose H, Obagi ZE, Laub DR. Obagi's modified trichloroacetic acid (TCA)-controlled variable-depth peel: a study of clinical signs correlating with histological findings. Ann Plast Surg. 1996; 36(3):225–237

[4] O'Connor AA, et al. Chemical peels: A review of current practice. Australas J Dermatol. 2017

19 Maximizing Safety with Radiofrequency-Based Devices

Erez Dayan and Rod J. Rohrich

Abstract

Radiofrequency (RF) energy delivered internally or externally has been successfully used to treat rhytids, jowling, skin laxity, telangiectasias, and other age-related skin changes. It has also been used to target subcutaneous tissues for subdermal adipose remodeling and contouring. RF devices create alternating currents to polarize tissue within an electrical path using negatively and positively charged electrodes to generate heat. Safe and consistent use of this technology depends on an understanding of (1) specific characteristics of the patient's skin and soft-tissue anatomy, (2) characteristics of the radiofrequency device, and (3) energy/tissue interactions. In this chapter, we outline the utility of radiofrequency technology, including indications, contraindications, and anatomic danger zones.

Keywords: facial contouring, skin tightening, radiofrequency, microneedle radiofrequency, catheter based radiofrequency

Key Points

- RF is of particular interest as a safe and effective way to decrease skin laxity in facial rejuvenation; either as a primary treatment or to correct recurrent laxity after a facelift or neck lift (▶ **Fig. 19.1**).[1,2,3]
- Thermal devices such as those that are radiofrequency (RF)-based impact the soft tissues at a molecular level by collagen denaturation at 55 to 60°C, leading to subsequent neocollagenesis, ellastogenesis, angiogenesis, and subdermal adipose remodeling over the subsequent 4 to 8 weeks from treatment (**Video 19.1**).[2,4,5]
- RF energy can be delivered using monopolar, bipolar, or multipolar devices. Other variants of RF delivery include fractional, sublative, and combination technologies (laser, light, electromagnetic energy).[4,6,7,8,9]
- RF can be used safely in patients of all skin types, and is most effective in younger patients with mild skin laxity and good skin elasticity.[2,3,10]
- Frequently, RF is used in conjunction with liposuction. RF energy is applied first to tighten the fibroseptal network and induce skin tightening, while the subsequent liposuction decreases the underlying adipose tissue volume.[2,4,5,11]

19.1 Safety Considerations

- Unlike laser energy with selective photothermolysis, RF heating is nonselective. Thus, RF can be applied to any Fitzpatrick skin type without concern for damage to melanocytes or pigmentation changes. However, caution must be used to avoid thermal injury.
- Heating occurs either at the needle tip or along the entirety of the cannula, depending on whether the device is insulated or not.[2,4,9,11]
- Modern safety features include self-cooling RF technology (i.e., cryogen spray), internal/external temperature probes with shutdown features once predetermined target temperatures are reached, external

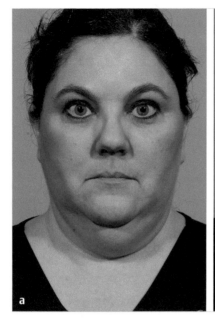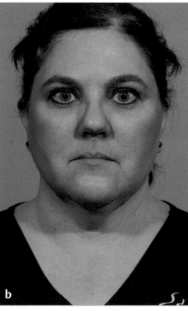

Fig. 19.1 (a) Pre- and (b) postoperative results after neck and jowl radiofrequency and liposuction.

near-infrared thermography cameras, and coated cannulas to avoid side and end hits.[2,3,11,12]

- A systematic approach of gradual heating should be applied to sequential areas in order to allow for efficient heating and to avoid burns/full-thickness skin injury.
- In cannula-based devices, heating is applied incrementally from deep to more superficial areas. One should avoid too many passes in one area. No more than 1 to 3 minutes in one particular area is recommended once the target temperature is reached.[2,11]

19.2 Pertinent Anatomy

19.2.1 Treatment Zones (▶Fig. 19.2):

1. Lower third of the face and neck.
2. Midneck.
3. Lateral neck.
4. Jowls.

19.2.2 Nontreatment Zones (▶Fig. 19.2):

1. Mid/Upper face.
2. Marrionette lines.
3. Forehead.
4. Perioral/periorbital areas.

19.2.3 Marginal Mandibular Nerve Anatomy[13]:

- The marginal mandibular branch of the facial nerve passes beneath the platysma and depressor anguli oris, supplying muscles of the lower lip and chin (▶**Fig. 19.3**).
- The marginal mandibular branch of the facial nerve is found superficial to the facial artery and anterior to the facial vein.

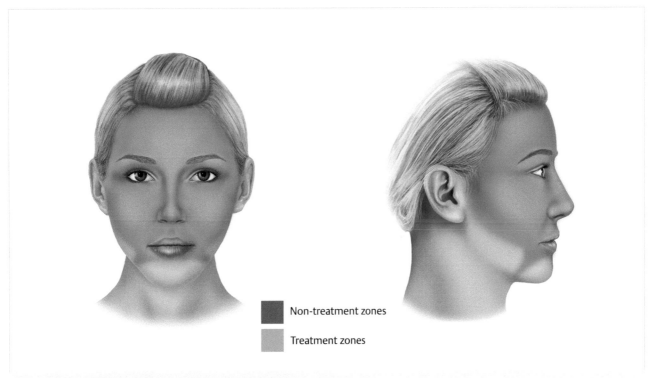

Non-treatment zones

Treatment zones

Fig. 19.2 Treatment and nontreatment radiofrequency zones.

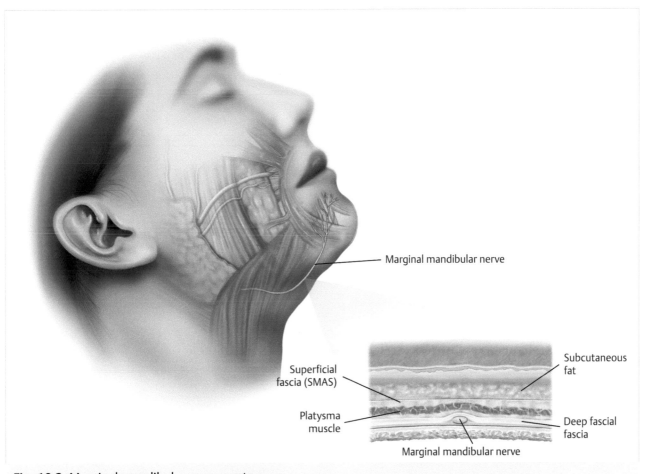

Marginal mandibular nerve

Superficial
fascia (SMAS)

Subcutaneous
fat

Platysma
muscle

Deep fascial
fascia

Marginal mandibular nerve

Fig. 19.3 Marginal mandibular nerve anatomy.

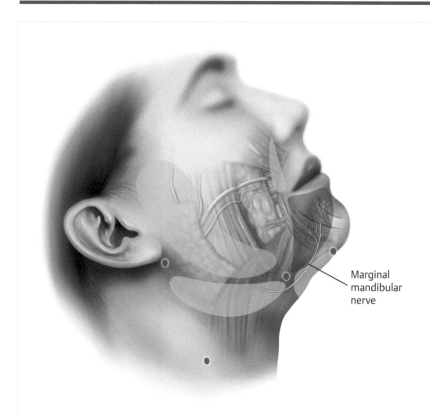

Fig. 19.4 Access ports placement to avoid marginal mandibular and mental nerve injury.

Marginal
mandibular
nerve

- Entry ports for RF cannulas should be designed to allow for radial motion away from the most superficial area of the marginal mandibular nerve (midmandible, 2 cm posterior to the oral commissure, beneath superficial musculoaponeurotic system [SMAS]) and mental nerve (midmandible below second premolar anterior to SMAS) (▶ **Fig. 19.4**).

19.2.4 Mental Nerve[14]

- A branch of the inferior alveolar nerve (CN V) which provides sensation to the anterior chin and lower lip as well as the intervening gingivae.
- The nerve emerges at the mental foramen in the mandible and travels beneath the depressor anguli oris muscle into three branches (the skin of the chin and the skin and mucous membrane of the lower lip).

19.3 Technical Points

- Most common inadvertent targets include superficial sensory nerves and the marginal mandibular nerve as it approximates areas of jowling and soft-tissue descent at the border of the mandible.[1,3]
- RF probe should remain subcutaneous at all times, and should never be beneath platysma or an SMAS layer.
- A radial motion is used with energy application only on withdrawal.
- Stop energy application 1 cm prior to access point as to not apply energy recurrently when the probe moves proximally.
- Tumescent injection allows for hydrodissection above the platysma/SMAS layer to avoid inadvertent subplatysmal cannula placement.

References

[1] Blugerman G, Schavelzon D, Paul MD. A safety and feasibility study of a novel radiofrequency-assisted liposuction technique. Plast Reconstr Surg. 2010; 125(3):998–1006

[2] Chia CT, Theodorou SJ, Hoyos AE, Pitman GH. Radiofrequency-Assisted Liposuction Compared with Aggressive Superficial, Subdermal Liposuction of the Arms: A Bilateral Quantitative Comparison. Plast Reconstr Surg Glob Open. 2015; 3(7):e459

[3] Gentile RD, Kinney BM, Sadick NS. Radiofrequency Technology in Face and Neck Rejuvenation. Facial Plast Surg Clin North Am. 2018; 26(2):123–134

[4] Sadick N, Rothaus KO. Aesthetic Applications of Radiofrequency Devices. Clin Plast Surg. 2016; 43(3):557–565

[5] Swanson E. Does Radiofrequency Assistance Improve Skin Contraction after Liposuction? Plast Reconstr Surg Glob Open. 2015; 3(10):e545

[6] Kao HK, Li Q, Flynn B, et al. Collagen synthesis modulated in wounds treated by pulsed radiofrequency energy. Plast Reconstr Surg. 2013; 131(4):490e–498e

[7] Levy AS, Grant RT, Rothaus KO. Radiofrequency Physics for Minimally Invasive Aesthetic Surgery. Clin Plast Surg. 2016; 43(3):551–556

[8] Li Q, Kao H, Matros E, Peng C, Murphy GF, Guo L. Pulsed radiofrequency energy accelerates wound healing in diabetic mice. Plast Reconstr Surg. 2011; 127(6):2255–2262

[9] Pritzker RN, Robinson DM. Updates in noninvasive and minimally invasive skin tightening. Semin Cutan Med Surg. 2014; 33(4):182–187

[10] Chen B, Kao HK, Dong Z, Jiang Z, Guo L. Complementary Effects of Negative-Pressure Wound Therapy and Pulsed Radiofrequency Energy on Cutaneous Wound Healing in Diabetic Mice. Plast Reconstr Surg. 2017; 139(1):105–117

[11] Theodorou S, Chia C. Radiofrequency-assisted Liposuction for Arm Contouring: Technique under Local Anesthesia. Plast Reconstr Surg Glob Open. 2013; 1(5):e37

[12] Keramidas E, Rodopoulou S. Radiofrequency-assisted Liposuction for Neck and Lower Face Adipodermal Remodeling and Contouring. Plast Reconstr Surg Glob Open. 2016; 4(8):e850

[13] Balagopal PG, George NA, Sebastian P. Anatomic variations of the marginal mandibular nerve. Indian J Surg Oncol. 2012; 3(1):8–11

[14] Betz D, Fane K. Nerve Block, Mental. In: StatPearls. 2018: Treasure Island (FL)

20 Maximizing Safety with Cryolipolysis

Erez Dayan and Rod J. Rohrich

Abstract

Cryolipolysis is among the most popular noninvasive treatments for focal adipose excess. The FDA cleared cryolipolysis for reduction of fat deposits in the flanks, abdomen, and thighs between 2010 and 2014; this technology has since emerged as a leader among noninvasive body contouring devices. Cryolipolysis works by preferentially destroying fat cells through a controlled thermal reduction. Exposure to below normal, but above-freezing temperature induces apoptosis of fat cells and takes advantage of adipocyte sensitivity to the cooling process when compared to surrounding tissues.

Keywords: cryolipolysis, noninvasive body contouring, adipocyte apoptosis, lipodystrophy

Key Points

- Cryolipolysis is based on the concept that lipid-rich tissues are more susceptible to cold injury than surrounding water-rich tissue (▶ **Fig. 20.1**).[1,2,3,4]
- The method involves controlled application of cooling within the temperature range of -11 to 5°C.[1,5,6]
- Cryolipolysis targets adipocytes while sparing skin, nerves, vessels, and muscles.[7]
- This technology appears to be safe in the short and long term. It has not been shown to have any effect on cholesterol, triglycerides, low-density lipoprotein, high-density lipoprotein, liver function (aspartate aminotransferase (AST)/alanine aminotransferase (ALT) bilirubin), albumin, or glucose.[7]
- The mechanism for cryolipolysis is not fully understood. Theories include adipocyte apoptosis by cellular edema, reduced Na-K-ATPase activity, elevated lactic acid levels, and mitochondrial free radical release. Ultimately, an inflammatory process leads to adipocyte death and removal by macrophages within 3 months.[8]
- Complications are rare and typically resolve a few weeks after treatment. Adverse events include erythema, bruising, swelling, sensitivity, and pain. No persistent ulcerations, scarring, paresthesias, hematomas, blistering, bleeding, hyperpigmentation/hypopigmentation, or infections have been described.[8,9,10]
- Few isolated case reports have described paradoxical adipose hyperplasia after cryolipolysis treatment (est 1:20,000).[11,12,13,14,15]

20.1 Safety Considerations

- Ideal candidates are patients who require small focal areas of adipose tissue removal. Patients with excess adipose tissue or skin must be appropriately counselled, as they are likely better candidates for liposuction or excisional operations.
- Contraindications to cryolipolysis include cold-induced conditions such as cryoglobinemia, cold urticarial, and paroxysmal cold hemoglobinuria.[8,16]
- Cryolipolysis should not be performed in treatment areas with severe varicose veins, dermatitis, or other cutaneous lesions.[8,16]

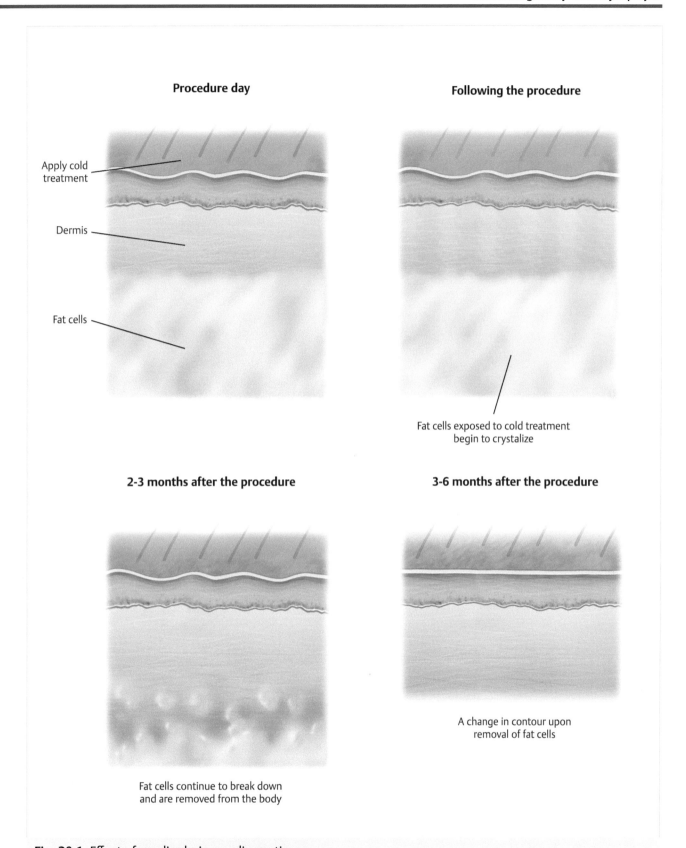

Fig. 20.1 Effect of cryolipolysis on adipose tissue.

20.2 Clinical Correlations

- Cryolipolysis has been shown to safely and effectively reduce subcutaneous fat and has FDA clearance for treatment of the flanks, abdomen, thighs, submental area, back, bra area, underneath the buttocks, and the arm.
- Treatment protocols have yet to be optimized to maximize results. Patients should be notified that multiple treatments are often required for the desired effect.
- Subsequent treatments lead to further fat reduction; however, the extent of improvement has not been shown to be as dramatic as the first treatment. There are also variations to the degree of improvement with additional treatments based on the anatomic site (i.e., subsequent treatments of the abdomen have more marked results when compared to the flanks).[7,8]
- Massage/kneading of the soft tissues posttreatment has been shown to improve the efficacy of cryolipolysis clinically and histologically.[8,17]

References

[1] Kilmer SL, Burns AJ, Zelickson BD. Safety and efficacy of cryolipolysis for non-invasive reduction of submental fat. Lasers Surg Med. 2016; 48(1):3–13

[2] Leal Silva H, Carmona Hernandez E, Grijalva Vazquez M, Leal Delgado S, Perez Blanco A. Noninvasive submental fat reduction using colder cryolipolysis. J Cosmet Dermatol. 2017; 16(4):460–465

[3] Lee SJ, Jang HW, Kim H, Suh DH, Ryu HJ. Non-invasive cryolipolysis to reduce subcutaneous fat in the arms. J Cosmet Laser Ther. 2016; 18(3):126–129

[4] Meyer PF, da Silva RM, Oliveira G, et al. Effects of Cryolipolysis on Abdominal Adiposity. Case Rep Dermatol Med. 2016; 2016:6052194

[5] Li MK, Mazur C, DaSilva D, Canfield D, McDaniel DH. Use of 3-Dimensional Imaging in Submental Fat Reduction After Cryolipolysis. Dermatol Surg. 2018; 44(6):889–892

[6] Wanitphakdeedecha R, Sathaworawong A, Manuskiatti W. The efficacy of cryolipolysis treatment on arms and inner thighs. Lasers Med Sci. 2015; 30(8):2165–2169

[7] Bernstein EF. Long-term efficacy follow-up on two cryolipolysis case studies: 6 and 9 years post-treatment. J Cosmet Dermatol. 2016; 15(4):561–564

[8] Ingargiola MJ, Motakef S, Chung MT, Vasconez HC, Sasaki GH. Cryolipolysis for fat reduction and body contouring: safety and efficacy of current treatment paradigms. Plast Reconstr Surg. 2015; 135(6):1581–1590

[9] Jeong SY, Kwon TR, Seok J, Park KY, Kim BJ. Non-invasive tumescent cryolipolysis using a new 4D handpiece: a comparative study with a porcine model. Skin Res Technol. 2017; 23(1):79–87

[10] Jones IT, Vanaman Wilson MJ, Guiha I, Wu DC, Goldman MP. A split-body study evaluating the efficacy of a conformable surface cryolipolysis applicator for the treatment of male pseudogynecomastia. Lasers Surg Med. 2018

[11] Ho D, Jagdeo J. A Systematic Review of Paradoxical Adipose Hyperplasia (PAH) Post-Cryolipolysis. J Drugs Dermatol. 2017; 16(1):62–67

[12] Karcher C, Katz B, Sadick N. Paradoxical Hyperplasia Post Cryolipolysis and Management. Dermatol Surg. 2017; 43(3):467–470

[13] Keaney TC, Naga LI. Men at risk for paradoxical adipose hyperplasia after cryolipolysis. J Cosmet Dermatol. 2016; 15(4):575–577

[14] Kelly E, Rodriguez-Feliz J, Kelly ME. Paradoxical Adipose Hyperplasia after Cryolipolysis: A Report on Incidence and Common Factors Identified in 510 Patients. Plast Reconstr Surg. 2016; 137(3):639e–640e

[15] Kelly ME, Rodríguez-Feliz J, Torres C, Kelly E. Treatment of Paradoxical Adipose Hyperplasia following Cryolipolysis: A Single-Center Experience. Plast Reconstr Surg. 2018; 142(1):17e–22e

[16] Sasaki GH. Reply: Cryolipolysis for Fat Reduction and Body Contouring: Safety and Efficacy of Current Treatment Paradigms. Plast Reconstr Surg. 2016; 137(3):640e–641e

[17] Carruthers JD, Humphrey S, Rivers JK. Cryolipolysis for Reduction of Arm Fat: Safety and Efficacy of a Prototype CoolCup Applicator With Flat Contour. Dermatol Surg. 2017; 43(7):940–949

21 Maximizing Safety with Microneedling

Erez Dayan, David Dwayne Weir, Rod J. Rohrich, and E. Victor Ross

Abstract

Initially used in the treatment of scars, microneedling has been in use since the early 1990s. Since then, microneedling (once referred to as collagen induction therapy) has become a popular minimally invasive procedure for skin rejuvenation. Microneedles are used to penetrate the dermis and lead to percutaneous collagen, elastin, and capillary induction/reorganization. The needles used are on the order of microns, with needle length ranging from 0.5 to 1.5 mm. Microneedling can also work in synergy with a variety of drugs to augment transdermal delivery through micropores, among the most popular of which is platelet-rich plasma (PRP).

Keywords: microneedling, percutaneous collagen induction, facial rejuventation, platelet rich plasma

Key Points

- Microneedling penetrates the dermis and initiates the body's inflammatory and healing cascades, thus inducing a fluctuation of growth factors (FGF, TGF, and PDF) resulting in fibroblast activation and neocollagenesis, elastogenesis, and angiogenesis.[1,2,3]
- Within a week of microneedling, a fibronectin matrix scaffold develops, over which collagen organizes, ultimately leading to skin tightening.[3,4,5]
- Microneedling has been used successfully to treat acne scarring, nonacne scarring, hyperpigmentation, alopecia, and hyperhidrosis, as well as being used as a drug delivery technique.[2,3,4,5,6,7,8]
- Microneedling devices come in a variety of needle arrangements (e.g., tattoo devices, rollers, electronic devices) and materials (glass, silicone, metals, biodegradable polymers). The most commonly used methods for microneedling include rollers and electronic devices.

21.1 Safety Considerations

- There is only one FDA-approved microneedling device currently on the U.S. market (SkinPen [Bellus Medical]).
- The only FDA-approved use of microneedling is for atrophic scarring of the face (excluding within orbital rim).
- SkinPen can be used in face/neck/body areas and is off label for use within the orbital rim. There are several different microneedling devices currently in practice, with a wide variety of needle quality and safety features. The SkinPen is the first to offer quality control research and data confirming their disposable needling tip device's safety and quality.
- Cross contamination of needles, and in turn bodily fluids, must be carefully controlled. Ideally, the microneedling device used should have a sealed hand-piece with a disposable microneedling unit for one-time use only. When combined with PRP, utmost care must be taken to systematically organize plasma and not inadvertently mix among patients.

- Varying methods of anesthetic, including over-the-counter topical anesthetics, as well as specialty compounded formulations, are used to minimize patient discomfort. Under the direct supervision of a qualified medical provider, compounded topical formulations of analgesics can be used with caution. In our practice, when performing microneedling on multiple treatment areas, a staggering multistep approach with topical anesthetics is used to avoid lidocaine toxicity.
- Cases of granulomas have been reported, particularly when using nonsterile preparations, topically in conjunction with micro needling. Ideally, only sterile products that are manufactured to be delivered intradermally should be applied on the surface when performing microneedling.
- Needle depth can range from 0.25 mm to 3 mm depending on the device. An understanding of the anatomy of the treatment area is necessary to determine the safety of the needle depth.[1,2,7] Similar to chemical peel and laser safety, certain treatment areas are treated with a deeper depth of microneedling, while other treatment areas are treated with a shallower depth of needle penetration (▶ **Fig. 21.1**) (**Video 21.1**).[3,9,10]
- Devices that offer deeper microneedling settings (1.5 mm–3.0 mm) must be used with caution, particularly in patients with thin skin, as deeper needles (> 3mm) can cause sensory nerve damage.

21.2 Safe Zones

- Areas that offer the most underlying fat and a thick dermis are considered more safe zones. These areas include the zygomatic region, buccal region, perioral region, mental region, and the parotid-masseteric region.

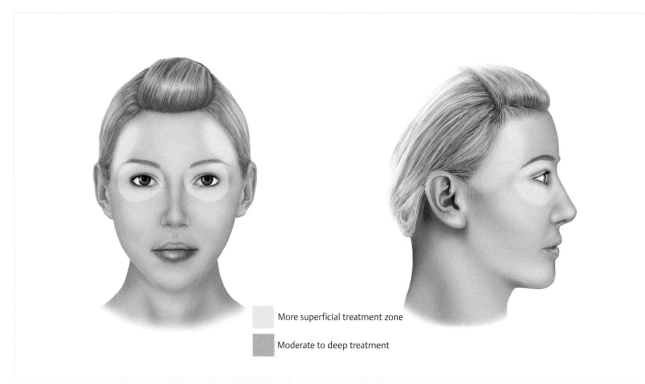

More superficial treatment zone

Moderate to deep treatment

Fig. 21.1 Deep and superficial treatment zones for microneedling.

21.3 Transitional Zones

- Transitional zones tend to have thinner underlying fat and a thinner dermis; these include the temporal region, the infraorbital region, the neck region, and the frontal region.

21.4 Danger Zones

- Danger zones based on the underling skin structure include within the orbital rim and the perioral region. (Conservative treatment is applied, typically 0.25mm depth)

21.5 Clinical Correlations

- Microneedling can be used in all Fitzpatrick skin types.
- There is no heat component to standard microneedling, so concern over burns, scarring, or pigmentation changes is virtually eliminated.

21.6 Technical Points

- Three different motions are applied per area: vertical, horizontal, and circular.
- Stay perpendicular to the skin.
- Allow the device to do the work; do not apply excess pressure, and do not drag the device across the skin.

References

[1] Ablon G. Safety and Effectiveness of an Automated Microneedling Device in Improving the Signs of Aging Skin. J Clin Aesthet Dermatol. 2018; 11(8):29–34

[2] Duncan DI. Microneedling with Biologicals: Advantages and Limitations. Facial Plast Surg Clin North Am. 2018; 26(4):447–454

[3] Food and Drug Administration, HHS. Medical Devices; General and Plastic Surgery Devices; Classification of the Microneedling Device for Aesthetic Use. Final order. Fed Regist. 2018; 83(111):26575–26577

[4] Mazzella C, Cantelli M, Nappa P, Annunziata MC, Delfino M, Fabbrocini G. Confocal microscopy can assess the efficacy of combined microneedling and skinbooster for striae rubrae. J Cosmet Laser Ther. 2018; •••:1–4

[5] Zduńska K, Kołodziejczak A, Rotsztejn H. Is skin microneedling a good alternative method of various skin defects removal. Dermatol Ther (Heidelb). 2018; 31(6):e12714

[6] Al Qarqaz F, Al-Yousef A. Skin microneedling for acne scars associated with pigmentation in patients with dark skin. J Cosmet Dermatol. 2018; 17(3):390–395

[7] Badran KW, Nabili V. Lasers, Microneedling, and Platelet-Rich Plasma for Skin Rejuvenation and Repair. Facial Plast Surg Clin North Am. 2018; 26(4):455–468

[8] Sezgin B, Özmen S. Fat grafting to the face with adjunctive microneedling: a simple technique with high patient satisfaction. Turk J Med Sci. 2018; 48(3):592–601

[9] Schmitt L, Marquardt Y, Amann P, et al. Comprehensive molecular characterization of microneedling therapy in a human three-dimensional skin model. PLoS One. 2018; 13(9):e0204318

[10] Soliman M, Mohsen Soliman M, El-Tawdy A, Shorbagy HS. Efficacy of fractional carbon dioxide laser versus microneedling in the treatment of striae distensae. J Cosmet Laser Ther. 2018; •••:1–8

Index

Note: Page numbers set in **bold** or *italic* indicate headings or figures, respectively.